Cancer, Autism and Their Epigenetic Roots

K. John Morrow, Jr.

MCFARLAND HEALTH TOPICS
Series Editor Elaine A. Moore

McFarland & Company, Inc., Publishers
Jefferson, North Carolina

LIBRARY OF CONGRESS CATALOGUING-IN-PUBLICATION DATA

Morrow, John, 1938– author.
    Cancer, autism and their epigenetic roots / K. John Morrow, Jr.
      p.   cm. — (Mcfarland health topics)
    [Elaine A. Moore, series editor]
    Includes bibliographical references and index.

    ISBN 978-0-7864-7920-7 (softcover : acid free paper) ∞
    ISBN 978-1-4766-1563-9 (ebook)

    I. Title. II. Series: McFarland health topics.
[DNLM: 1. Epigenesis, Genetic. 2. Genetic Predisposition
to Disease. 3. Child Development Disorders, Pervasive—
genetics. 4. Neoplasms—genetics. QU 477]
  RB155.5   616'.042—dc23   2014016719

BRITISH LIBRARY CATALOGUING DATA ARE AVAILABLE

Front cover: Medical laboratory © iStock/Thinkstock

Printed in the United States of America

McFarland & Company, Inc., Publishers
  Box 611, Jefferson, North Carolina 28640
    www.mcfarlandpub.com

Acknowledgments

Epigenetics is an unusually complex, rapidly changing discipline. It is impossible to cover every aspect of this field, and new information is being added constantly, so that any description will be out of date by the time it is available to the reader. My goal was to give a very broad overview of this field, in a readable format. I have not provided details on many of the elegant representations of the precise modes of action of epigenetic signals. There are many fine reviews of this material that are accessible to both professional scientists and to general readers. Rather I have tried to present the scope of the field and its social and political ramifications. Inevitably, this involves simplifying and leaving out material. Since this is not intended as a scientific review of the field, it is not comprehensive, and in many cases I have greatly condensed or omitted complicated scientific models.

Furthermore, I have added at numerous points in the chapter notes information which I believe will amuse and inform the reader. However, many of these are tangential, and readers focused on the nature of epigenetics can pick and choose among these.

I have been very fortunate that many of the outstanding investigators and scientists in epigenetics and related disciplines have offered their time and critical abilities in reviewing this manuscript. However, I have drawn my own conclusions and made my own policy recommendations in the final chapters. These are my own opinions. Any errors or omissions in this book are strictly my own.

My thanks go out to Dr. Dean Edwards, Dr. Mike Skinner, Dr. Shuk-Mei Ho, Dr. John McCarrey, Dr. Heather Patisaul, Dr. Dana Dolinoy, and Dr. Wilber Baker, who have read and critiqued various sections of this manuscript. Dr. Douglas Stocco was especially helpful in introducing me to a number of these individuals.

Acknowledgments

Special thanks to Dr. Tesseny Sandgathe, who provided many useful comments and suggestions, and to Elise Morrow and Garima Naredi, whose artistic talents are seen in a number of the drawings and figures that accompany the manuscript.

My close friend, mystery writer Jack Kerley, gave me encouragement and writing suggestions and helped me wend my way through the literary jungle to find an agent.

That agent is Lisa Hagan who is one of my major fans. Her many thoughts and comments encouraged me to move forward with the book. And she led me to my publisher and its "Health Topics" series and series editor Elaine A. Moore.

And finally to Julie, who has supported and encouraged me on this journey for so many years.

Table of Contents

Preface: A Scientific Detective Story

This book is a personal scientific detective story delving into the exploding frequencies of a group of mental diseases affecting large segments of our society: autism, Alzheimer's disease, schizophrenia and bipolar disorders among many others. But there's more: an ugly collection of physical ailments, including cancer, the most carefully studied, diabetes and heart disease, just for starters.

It has long been assumed that those who were stricken with these diseases owed their fate to an unlucky combination of genes and environment. But in recent years a third player in this dance has been identified. This contributor was so ignored that twenty years ago even most biologists hardly gave it a second thought.

All this is changing now, as we welcome you to the world of *epigenetics*. While the term has a certain exotic air and high-tech sound to it, it is not a difficult concept, and it opens up a new level of understanding of the fundamental origins of health and sickness.

Basically put: As the incidence of these illnesses has ramped up, so has the exposure of the population to a witches' brew of pesticides, plasticizers, cosmetics and industrial chemicals. Other sources of concern are produced through industrial processes, such as heavy metals, petroleum products and radiation. Many of these substances are known to affect the behavior of genes through epigenetic routes. And now evidence is piling up, connecting exposure to them with the ascendency of these diseases.

I have written this book because I believe there is a wealth of evidence demonstrating that epigenetic mechanisms play a critical, and previously unrecognized, role in driving many of these diseases. In this unfolding story I will lay out the evidence and offer a course of action to slow and reverse this epidemic.

If our society takes imprudent action to limit this damage, we may run the risks of overreacting, squandering money and resources, and strangling economic growth. But time is running out. If we do not act with the knowledge that we have available, the consequences could be much worse: an unsupportable burden of disease and misery affecting individuals and society for generations to come.

My original intent in writing this book was to present a brief and topical review of the science of epigenetics, with special attention given to issues of health and disease. As I moved along in the writing, time after time I felt that it was necessary to add explanatory information as well as detailed references. But I didn't want to interrupt the flow of the book or allow the main message to get lost in the details. Many of these concepts and ideas that I encountered along the way are of great interest to general audiences and could constitute material for entire books in their own right.

I also wanted to share with readers some personal thoughts of my own, recollections and views about science and its practice today.

So the book can be read on two levels: first as a short exposition of the scientific, social and political issues raised by epigenetics, and second as a source for additional details on the scientific and social issues, as a supplement covering many ancillary topics.

I will post additional information on my website as it comes available (www.newportbiotech.com).

Introduction:
The 40-Year-Old Mystery

The cells just weren't behaving that day. It was 1973, and I was a faculty member at a university, with a brand new research program up and running. I'd been trained in genetics, and the premise of my research was that if we could apply techniques to mammalian cells that had been so successful in the study of bacterial genes, we could make big contributions to our understanding of heredity in mammals, especially humans.

We grew cells in glass bottles, covered with a fluid medium, much like blood, that nourished them, a technique known as cell culture. The cells came from tumors or embryonic tissues, so they weren't really normal body cells, but rather something that had been changed and adapted to life in an incubator, a process known as transformation. As they accustomed themselves to their new life they grew, divided and grew again, contentedly going on about their lives for as long as we would provide the cozy conditions that allowed them to flourish.

But here we were measuring variability in cultured cells, looking at how frequently they became resistant to anti-cancer drugs. We reasoned that if we could understand this process we could control it, and in the long run prevent cancers from becoming resistant to anti-cancer agents. But that day things weren't working out the way we had predicted, and I couldn't come up with a reasonable explanation.

Ordinarily, genes are pretty stable; they have to be. Living creatures couldn't exist if their hereditary material broke down and was reassembled in every generation. On the other hand, if genes, DNA, were completely stable and never shifted, then evolution couldn't take place. This is a fundamental premise of the theory of evolution, that natural selection acts by eliminating unsuitable variability from the population, and retaining the owners of successful genes.

3

So what's too much or too little variability? You can't say for sure. It depends on the particular set of conditions, but it was known at the time that mutations for well-known genetic diseases, like hemophilia, occurred in human populations about one time in a million. These mutations are changes in the DNA bases, and even in the 1970s, were well understood.

But the numbers we were getting from our miscreant cells were 10,000 times as high, numbers like one in a hundred! That means that if we tested 100 cells, one of them would turn out to be resistant to the anti-cancer drug we were examining. While this goes a long way to explaining why cancer patients so frequently experience resistance to chemotherapy in their tumors, it didn't help us understand how this resistance came about in the first place. These numbers were so high they seemed like an anomaly, something that didn't fit in with our concept of how genes should behave.

I had many conversations with the research group that I had assembled and we finally decided to write up the work and submit it to a specialized journal of cell biology. In the discussion section of the paper we suggested possible explanations, but there was no way we could test them. At that time some of the best scientists in the world were just beginning to take genes apart and clone DNA, and the human genome project was 25 years in the future. So we were at a dead end for this project.

But years later, I was writing a research report, reviewing new advances in genetics. In the course of this enterprise I did a lot of reading on epigenetics and I talked to many of the scientists who are on the forefront of epigenetics research. And the more I learned, the more worried I became.

With a fresh understanding of genes and the ability to take them apart and analyze them, a new branch of genetics has flowered, and I believe it explains my own mystery, but much more importantly, it opens up a whole new realm of science, with a vast new world of exciting possibilities on the one hand, yet terrifying threats to our survival on the other.

Epigenetics is a branch of the science of heredity which has been around for a long time, but until recently the tools to understand it were not available. It concerns the modification of genes, stretches of DNA, by chemical additions to the DNA molecule, not by changing the code letters. Epigenetic modification can be rapid and highly reversible, since one is modifying chemical groups that attach to DNA, not the code of DNA itself. We'll have more to say about that later, but let's consider why I speak of challenges and threats in the same sentence.

Challenges: If the concept of epigenetics offers an explanation for why genes can be so unstable, then it should be possible to block this instability, and control cancer, clamp down on the disorder and put the genie back in the bottle. By the same token, if epigenetic changes to genes are responsible for all or part of diseases such as autism, then it should also be possible to prevent this from happening by blocking access of the DNA to chemicals that might affect the genes involved.

Threats: But here's where the story becomes ugly and frightening. Because if these chemicals in our environment could change genes 10,000 times faster than they ordinarily would, doesn't this constitute a grave risk to our society? Doesn't this at least suggest that the phenomenal rise in the incidence of many diseases is driven by epigenetic changes?

Both the challenges and the threats are very real. What you will read here is a detective story, an investigation of epigenetics. We'll see what it is, how it works and why the scientific community did not pursue it until recently. You will find why many scientists believe that through epigenetics there is hope for a better, healthier world, an understanding of disease and a window to treatments for devastating diseases. At the same time you will learn the downside to these discoveries: the risk of environmental destruction and the building of a tsunami of illness brought about by our unwitting exposure to chemicals that cause epigenetic changes to our hereditary makeup.

And finally, we will see an answer to my 40-year-old medical mystery, how it links to epigenetics, and how these tools can be used to understand and control the damage caused by exposure to epigenetic chemicals. In doing so I will outline a roadmap to the future, that may offer hope to millions of families dealing with the ravages of diseases caused by exposure to these substances. While it may not be possible to completely eliminate epigenetic damage to our hereditary endowment, we will see that there are steps that can be taken to greatly reduce the risk to ourselves and our environment.

I cannot argue that confronting this problem will be easy, but I can say that not confronting it will be a terrible mistake.

1

The Long Winding Road
to the Long Neck

"It's all in the DNA!"

"The real reason for success or failure lies within—that is, in the culture of a company, says a new book!"[1]

How many times have we heard this "in the DNA" expression? We all know what it means. This cliché means that some pattern of speech or action or some way of thinking is absolutely entrenched in whoever or whatever we are talking about. It really doesn't mean that these marvelously successful companies have DNA molecules that are programmed to make super terrific products and consummate red hot business mergers. Or that some politician or public figure makes certain statements because they have these patterns hard-wired in some way into their genetic material, or chromosomes or genome.

We all know it means that some action or activity is consistent, will occur over and over again, is solid, fixed. The person or entity that we're talking has always done it, always will. Because that's what most people think of, when they think of DNA: it's solid, it's consistent, it doesn't change over time.

And on the whole they're correct. But aside from the obvious fact that inanimate objects don't have DNA, the expression doesn't make much sense, since it invariably refers to the way people act or speak or behave, and we all know these are learned or acquired patterns of behavior, so they couldn't possibly be programmed in the DNA.

But what if acquired traits could be inherited? What if it were possible (for example) for a person to suffer from a miserable environment, develop dysfunctional behavior, and then pass that behavior on, through his or her genes to the children and even to the grandchildren? In the past it was assumed that lousy parenting caused mistreated children to be lousy parents. And by and large, that's what usually happens. Dysfunctional people create a bad environment and aren't able to raise properly adjusted kids.

What I'm going to argue here is that in addition or at the same time, exposure to stress or certain chemicals, or a variety of other factors, could modify gene expression so that the exposed individual suffers a load of harm and that this damage is perpetuated and passed to subsequent generations.

This may seem an extravagant claim, and I wouldn't make it if there were not a strong body of scientific evidence to back it up. But we need to start at the beginning.

The French Connection

It may have been the best of times and the worst of times, but 18th century France was a good place and a good time to do science. Even though it didn't go smoothly for all French scientists (Lavoisier, the discoverer of oxygen, got his head lopped off[2] in the French Revolution), there was great intellectual ferment, and much of the foundation of modern science was laid down during this period. In addition to scientists who got their hands dirty in the laboratory there was much discussion in the salons, where intellectuals and groupies got together to discuss the latest philosophical topics of the day. When we think of this period, the names of Molière and Voltaire come to mind, as brilliant writers and philosophers. The work of the naturalist Georges Cuvier and his discovery of dinosaur remains was widely discussed. The French Revolution in 1789 slowed down the salon tradition, but scientific discovery continued.

By 1809 things had quieted down and Jean-Baptiste Pierre Antoine de Monet, Chevalier de la Marck (Lamarck) published his *Philosophie zoologique ou exposition des considérations relatives à l'histoire naturelle des animaux*. In his long and eventful life he put forth an early version of the theory of evolution, but today is more remembered for what he got wrong rather than what he got right.

Lamarck argued first that organs that were not used gradually disappeared over generations and that traits acquired by an individual in

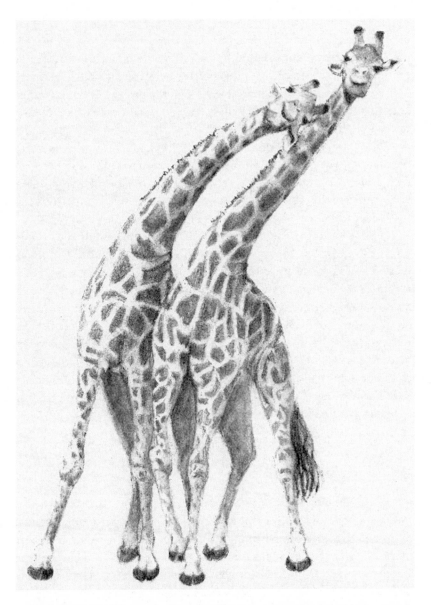

Figure 1. Giraffes sparring, another hypothesis for the evolution of the long neck. The classic explanation, formulated by Lamarck, was that the giraffe's long neck was the result of straining to reach the higher leaves, and this slightly strained and elongated neck was passed to the descendants. The modern theory posited that random mutations produced a range of progeny with different neck lengths, and those with the longer necks were more successful at obtaining food. They produced more offspring, and the long neck was spread through the population. Recently, however, other evolutionary biologists have argued that a long, powerful neck gives males an advantage as they spar for possession of the females. Drawing by Elise Morrow.

the course of its lifetime could be passed to the offspring. The classic example was the stretching of the giraffe's neck to reach the high leaves in the acacia trees on the African veldt, and the passing of this stretched neck to its offspring.[3] There are alternative explanations for the evolution of the long neck, as shown in Figure 1.

The unfortunate choice of the giraffe as Lamark's poster child for his theories was put to rest in the late 19th century, and is surely incorrect. Today we know that in the vast majority of cases, DNA is stable, variations in the DNA code occur rarely, beneficial mutations are retained, and adverse ones are eliminated in the battle for survival.

It's important to understand why Lamarck's reasoning didn't hold up. In the early 19th century there was not the vaguest notion of information storage or transfer within the cell. The microscope was a fairly rudimentary device, and no one had figured out how to preserve cells and stain them, in order to reveal them clearly under the microscope. So during this period one could propose mechanisms by which information (the stress of stretching the neck, say) would flow back to the place where information was stored, wherever that was. Then these data would be acted on, and in the next generation, the baby giraffes would have slightly longer necks. But this was all fairly mystical, and certainly not substantiated by any experimental proof.

DNA Takes the Day

We all know the story of Gregor Mendel, an obscure Augustinian monk, toiling away in his monastery garden with his pea plants. Mendel presented his work establishing the existence of genes to the members of the Natural Science Society in the town of Brno in Moravia (now the Czech Republic) in 1865. Historians of science have argued interminably over why such a clear and memorable scientific discovery was totally ignored for the next 35 years. Most agree that it wasn't because the scientists of that day were uninformed or too dense to appreciate what Mendel had done. Nor was it a case of simple arrogance, even though Mendel was hardly a member of the scientific establishment. But Mendel was highly educated for the time in which he lived, and had studied at the University of Vienna under the best scientists of the day.

Rather, the big stumbling block to the acceptance of what Mendel had accomplished was that he used a numerical analysis, which was not part of the way biologists looked at the world, and because science had not been able to identify anything that could carry these "genes" through cell divisions and distribute them to the next generation. Without such a mechanism, their existence appeared mystical and hypothetical.[4]

In the next few decades scientists in Germany and other countries discovered how to prepare tissues for clear viewing under the microscope with stains and fixatives that made the microscopic parts of the cells stand out. This revealed the existence of the cell nucleus and the chromosomes, which were parceled out equally in every cell division. They also saw that the chromosome number was halved in the egg and sperm cell and reestablished in the next generation. So by the end of the 19th century, it was clear that cells carried important packets, and these packages were the bearers of hereditary information.

When the concept of the gene was developed in the late 19th and early 20th century, the idea of the "inheritance of acquired characteristics" was put to rest. There appeared to be no way that information could feed back into the nucleus and affect the chromosomes, so the rule was laid down that information flowed in one direction, from the genes to the final product, plant or animal or bacterium. At this point the interaction of genes and environment wasn't even on the table, as not enough was known about it to bring it into the picture.

Thus the 20th century could be call the "century of the gene." From the 1950s on there was an avalanche of discoveries that filled in the gaps and holes in our notion of what genes are and how they operate. During this period, millions of scientific papers were published which built the picture of the gene as a piece of DNA composed of small molecules linked together in a spiral called a double helix. Along this spiral is an array of four similar molecules called bases. The arrangement of bases constitutes a code, and this code specifies the ordering of amino acids in the gene product, which is a protein. The information is transmitted to the cytoplasm by an intermediary, RNA, and the machinery of protein synthesis takes these instructions and assembles the proteins. So it was assumed that the flow of information went in one direction, from DNA to RNA to protein. This was the mantra that impressionable young minds such as my own learned during the early discovery phase of molecular biology.

The proteins are what make up our "phenotype," the overall representation of the individual. So these proteins do all the tasks that need to be done to make an entire, functioning creature. All of our organs, blood, brain, kidneys, skin, muscle are composed of special proteins, all coded for by different genes. So the genes are a compact code that specifies everything that will be in the final product.

Of course genes need to be turned on and off, and so genes that regulate other genes were discovered and described in detail. As gene sequencing grew from a slow, difficult process to a highly automated, extremely rapid technology, the amount of information expanded tremendously. Genetic instrumentation and molecular biology have advanced so far and so fast that you can have your entire genome sequenced for between $4,000 and $10,000. And it is predicted that the cost will soon drop to around $1,000.[5] This generates three billion bytes of information, and there is a great deal of uncertainty and confusion at this time as to what all this information does. Genetic counselors do not recommend that people get their genome sequenced for no particular reason, since there is still so much unknown about what all this DNA is trying to tell us.

The discoveries in genetics and molecular biology didn't leave much room for alternative ways of looking at our heredity. But as in any good detective story there were clues to a different narrative that were left about, ignored by the unwary. For a long time, since the mid 20th century, scientists had been wondering how the genes that control embryos switch on and off. Even then it was evident that there had to be some way of temporarily controlling their behavior, and a British embryologist, Conrad Waddington, applied the term "epigenetics" to this aspect of control.[6] Over time the term has come to mean any part of genetic expression that is not coded by the DNA. But no one was able to reconcile Waddington's ideas about embryos and how their genes are controlled with the prevailing notion that it was all wrapped up in the linear tape of the four bases or code letters (adenines, cytosines, guanines and thymines) that make up the DNA and are crammed into the chromosomes.

The emerging picture that scientists had constructed by the 1970s was dominated by the concept of the genetic language, the code carried in the DNA, as being the fundamental basis of heredity. And today that is what we learn in high school biology, and most popular expositions of genetics covered in the media use this as their starting point for whatever news from the genetics front that they are reporting.

Attack of the Clones

Perhaps one of the most misunderstood and overworked biological concepts that came out of the 1960s and 70s was the concept of "clones." The dictionary definition is straightforward: a "clone" is simply a member of a group of genetically identical individuals, produced naturally or by artificial means.[7] While it has been used over and over again as a science fiction motif, its relevance to epigenetics lies in what it revealed about how genes are controlled in the course of the development of an embryo.

When an egg is fertilized by a sperm, it begins to divide, and it forms a ball of cells, called a blastula, that are rather undistinguished at this youthful stage. The cells all look alike, they all have the same number of chromosomes, and if one measures various gene functions, they reveal no clue as to what these embryonic cells will eventually become. But later the developing embryo will start to produce the organs that will serve it in adulthood, and genes are turned on and off in these cells that make, say, brain proteins or liver proteins. So it must be that the unexpressed genes are not mutated or disposed of, but are there in a dormant state, and only wake up at the appropriate time. It was widely assumed that this process was irreversible, and once a cell differentiated into, say, a liver cell, there was no way that it could be turned around.

Moreover, the genes are controlled in such a way that different ones are activated in different organs. This process has been extensively studied over the years, and it is now known that hundreds, probably thousands of genes are turned on and turned off by epigenetic events in the course of the development of an embryo into a complete adult individual.

The exact timing and precise accuracy of these events mean that the period of embryonic and fetal development is a highly coordinated system, especially vulnerable to outside environmental effects.[8]

In the 1960s scientists working with frog embryos learned to manipulate the cells using a dissection microscope and glass needles. Amphibian cells are much larger than mammalian cells; this was what dictated the choice of frogs. It was done freehand, and required patience and skill, but with a lot of practice lab workers acquired the ability to move cells around and separate them from one another without destroying them. But what got the attention of the public was the fact that when the nuclei of cells from very young embryos were separated and physically forced into unfertilized frog eggs from which the egg cell nucleus had been removed, in at least some circumstances the manipulated eggs actually developed into normal frogs. This meant that from a single embryo, consisting of dozens of cells, you could theoretically make dozens of little frogs, and they should all be identical copies of one another. They would look alike, and their froggy personalities would be identical, at least to the extent that frogs do have unique personalities. From this point it wasn't much of a jump to imagine cloning being done in humans.

Much of this early work was done on *Rana catesbeiana*, the common bullfrog, by two embryologists working in Philadelphia, Robert Briggs and Thomas King.[9] I knew Thomas King in the 1960s when I was a postdoctoral fellow at the Institute for Cancer Research (now the Fox Chase Cancer Center) in Philadelphia. King always appeared to me to be somewhat morose, I suspect because at that time, the work that he and Briggs had accomplished had not garnered them wider recognition, such as a Nobel Prize. He eventually bowed out of laboratory science and left the institute for an administrative position at the National Institutes of Health in Bethesda.

Other scientists took up the effort, the most successful being John Gurdon, who days before the time of this writing received the Nobel Prize (both Briggs and King have long since died, and so could not be considered). Gurdon used a different frog, known as Xenopus, and made numerous changes in the lab protocol. As Gurdon labored away, the frequency of successful nuclear transfers (as they came to be called) became greater and greater. Finally Gurdon found that it was even possible to take much later stage embryos, remove a cell from the gut that was already making gut functions, and move it into a frog egg without its own nucleus, activate it, and eventually recover a fully formed, normal frog. Within a few years it became a standard procedure for studying amphibian development, and a number of noteworthy scientific discoveries were accomplished.[10]

So now all the pieces of the cloning machine were in place. It was indeed within the realm of possibility to produce a normal, healthy animal from a mature body cell that could be turned around in its tracks and made to start all over again. But only in frogs.

The success of the nuclear transfer investigations produced a cottage industry of science fiction; books, movies, TV programs. There are many fictional books about cloning listed on the Internet, and most of them have not worn well over the years. Probably the most famous was *The Boys from Brazil*, in which the infamous Josef Mengele, hiding out in Paraguay, makes multiple copies of Hitler in the hopes of establishing a Fourth Reich. It was made into a film in 1978, and is probably the most successful attempt to bring the idea of cloning to the big screen. Featuring Gregory Peck, James Mason and a number of famous actors of that period, it was a dramatic and commercial success. It is notable for its convincing details, including a fascinating sequence in which an Austrian biologist explains to Nazi hunter Lawrence Olivier how rabbits and mice are cloned. The scene is complete with a lab film demonstrating how it is done, years before mammalian cloning was successfully accomplished. In another beautifully executed sequence, an aging Mengele fondly reminisces over his triumphant production of dozens of adorable baby Hitlers.

There are a multitude of other films, serious or silly. Designed to take advantage of the public's fascination with the concept, these themes were recycled as a plot device. During the science fiction craze, most scientists working in the field (myself included) did not believe that humans could be cloned or would ever be cloned. The cells were small and very easily damaged; there appeared to be no way that they could be manipulated without destroying them. Many scientists struggled late into the night trying to design a liquid medium that would keep the embryonic cells alive, achieving nothing but failure. Some scientists suggested that mammals were different and lacked the plasticity of frogs, unable to change their gene expression in mid flight.

In 1979 Karl Illmensee, a scientist at the University of Geneva, reported the successful cloning of three mice. I was invited by Illmensee to give a seminar in his department, and during my visit he told me of his success. I was stunned by his announcement, which he delivered in a matter of fact way, as if he were telling me that he had just found a bargain on tomatoes at the supermarket. That evening he and his colleagues took me to dinner at a Geneva restaurant where the wine and conversation flowed freely. Karl, however, was taciturn and withdrawn and left early. I assumed that he was so dedicated and obsessed with his investigations that he was returning to his lab for another round of experiments.

In the months and years following the publication of the paper,[11] the results were challenged by a member of his staff. An investigation by a university committee declared the work not to be fraudulent, but cited numerous errors and discrepancies. Illmensee eventually left the university in 1985, after there were reports that his colleagues recommended that his contract not be renewed. He found another academic position and despite the blot on his reputation, continued on in his career. He is still active today in human fertility research and is a scientist at a fertility treatment clinic in Patras, Greece. I corresponded with him recently during the preparation of this book, and he indicated that he did not wish to discuss this period of his life.

Despite the odd twists in this story, years later it turned out that mammals can be cloned. In 1997 Dr. Ian Wilmut and his colleagues at the University of Edinburgh succeeded in producing a viable, healthy sheep, the famous "Dolly," from a mammary gland cell of a mature ewe. This work marked the conclusion of years of hard work, but nobody ever claimed that research is easy (see Figure 2). Since that time, many different mammals have been successful targets of the "nuclear transfer" procedure. There are innumerable variations of this strategy, one of the most significant being the "transgenic mouse" protocol. In this approach, genes are inserted into mouse cells, and these cells combined with early mouse embryos, shown in Figure 3. Some of the embryos mature normally and produce patchwork animals that are a mix of the original cells and the cells with the foreign genes inserted into them.

Opposite: **Figure 2. The cloning of Dolly. The cloning of a sheep was a major triumph for the scientists at the Roslin Institute in Scotland. The procedure involves the isolation of an egg from one strain of sheep and removal of its nucleus. The egg, now lacking most of its genetic material, receives a cell from the mammary gland of another strain. After stimulation with a tiny electrical current, the egg is placed in a special culture fluid and begins to divide, forming an early stage known as a blastocyst. It is then introduced into a surrogate mother and allowed to proceed through a normal development. Every stage of the process is extremely challenging and required years of experimentation. Drawing by Garima Naredi.**

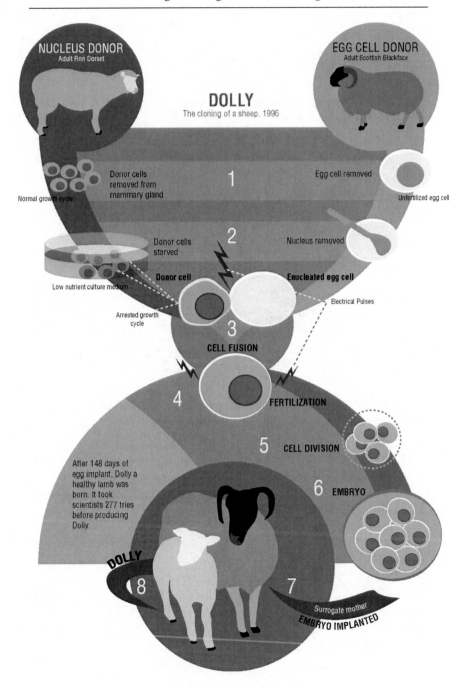

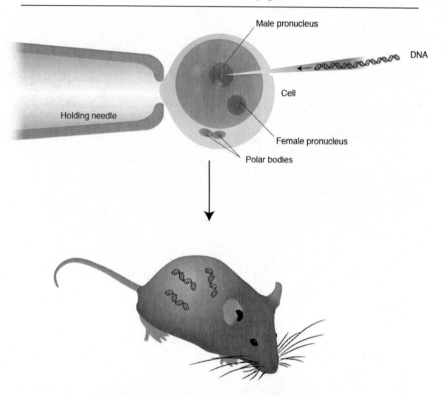

Figure 3. The making of a transgenic mouse. New technologies developed in recent decades have allowed the engineering of mice for a variety of research purposes. It is now possible to custom build strains of mice with human genes for a variety of traits, allowing the testing of drugs and many therapies without resort to primates or other expensive laboratory animals. Drawing by Garima Naredi.

When the Scottish researchers first succeeded in cloning mammals they were interested in the economic potential of producing identical lines of prize farm animals. The economic benefits turned out to be underwhelming. The technology was (and is) still challenging. The yields of viable embryos were low, which meant that many time-consuming and expensive procedures had to be carried out over and over again. A substantial proportion of the animals show various abnormalities and in numerous cases their overall health was poor. Today cloning of farm animals is looked upon as a means of retaining specific traits of value, and it is more of a research tool than a part of standard animal husbandry.[12]

Dolly was not a particularly robust specimen, and passed on to her reward at the age of six, whereas the normal lifespan for sheep is 12 years. There are other concerns that are still under investigation, and a company that Wilmut and his colleagues formed went belly up. However, the technology has been used in many studies on epigenetics, and has been widely and successfully applied in this area. We will have more to say about this in subsequent chapters.

This brief history of cloning would be incomplete without reference to the cloning debacle of Korean researcher Woo Suk Hwang in 2004–2006.[13] During this period, Hwang, a veterinarian researcher at the Seoul National University, achieved rock star status based on reports in prestigious journals that he had succeeded in establishing stem cell lines from human embryos, at that time a tremendous advance in human embryology, with major implication for disease treatments. Hwang's claim was that he had cloned a human blastocyst (a very early embryo and associated tissue consisting of about one hundred cells), through a process known as somatic cell nuclear transfer. This involved the insertion of a nucleus of a body (somatic) cell into a human egg. The Hwang claim was that they succeeded in getting the egg to divide to form a blastocyst, and from the cells of the blastocyst they were able to establish lines of embryonic stem cells. The 2005 paper reported the derivation of 11 human embryonic stem cell lines genetically matched to patients.

It turned out that there were massive irregularities and fraud on a very large scale. Hwang went from being the toast of Korean society to the depths of opprobrium. The Korean health sciences establishment is still picking up the pieces.[14]

As far as we know, humans have never been cloned, although there have been many unsupported claims to this effect. This idea is so rife with controversy and its benefits so limited that it is inconceivable that a legitimate private or public research group would ever attempt it. Which doesn't mean it isn't possible or that someone won't try.

To return to our story, the important point is that cloning experiments clearly show that by moving cells into different environments their genes can be turned on and off, over and over again. However, the early work didn't explain what was the force emanating from the egg cytoplasm that allowed a nucleus from a normal cell to direct the development of another whole, complete individual. At that time the question could not be answered, but with the passage of the years the question has been largely resolved, as we will see in later chapters.

Why Is There Fraud in Science?

If some of the pioneering work in epigenetics is so defaced by questionable research papers, why should we put any stock in this effort, and why do scientists fake results in the first place? We have no way of looking into the minds of people responsible for these acts, and it's not particularly useful to speculate. Without a doubt, cheating in science is the worst act of which a scientist can be guilty. It tears at the very fabric of trust that binds the scientific community together. There is nothing that can excuse it. There are always claims of immense pressure, desire for recognition, grants and promotions, and perhaps a feeling on the part of the fraudster that he knows the answer, and if he didn't get the experiments to work, it's just a matter of time, and he can go back and patch it up later. Mammalian cloning experiments are extremely difficult to carry out, even for the most able scientists, and it is likely that unscrupulous investigators think that they can get away with it because no one else has the skill to call them on it. It may take years for someone to develop the knowledge and technical skill to carry out cloning successfully.

But then, how much confidence can we have in these or any other scientific reports? Over the years there have been many accusations of scientific fraud, and there have been claims that it is widespread. Unfortunately, we really don't know, and any method of collecting evidence on such a charged and sensitive topic is fraught with difficulty.

But all scientists know the rules of the game. We have to be critical of any scientific paper, and the more important and ground-breaking the finding, the more critical we have to be. These are likely to be the bulk of questionable science, since it seems pointless to fake a trivial experiment, of no real value or impact.

In the final analysis, the answer is a utilitarian one. The fact that science works, that discoveries are repeatable, and lead to useful technologies, means that despite the fact that science, like any other human endeavor, is a flawed institution, it is not so flawed that it lacks the power to change our lives.

Epigenetics, the Rodney Dangerfield of Genetic Research

You might be wondering, if there were many indications back in the 1970s and 1980s that heredity was much more complex and nuanced, wasn't this concern picked up by the scientific community? Why wasn't there a call for more investigation? Why didn't the young field of epigenetics get more respect? Why didn't the detectives put the pieces of the puzzle together?

There is no simple answer to this question, but there are a number of factors that played into the lack of interest in epigenetics during this period.

First, scientists were just learning how to isolate genes and study them. Lab procedures that today can be carried out in minutes took days or weeks to accomplish.[15] The fundamentals of how epigenetic mechanisms cause genes to turn on and off were not understood. And the number of scientific papers on epigenetics was a dribble, just a handful per year. In contrast, the new techniques of gene analysis were pointed at the DNA, and exciting discoveries poured out in a vast torrent from laboratories all over the world.

Secondly, scientists are like everybody else—they may pride themselves on being original thinkers, but by and large, most scientists follow the herd. This isn't necessarily bad, since any scientific finding requires confirmation. An unimaginative, "me too" effort that confirms an important observation can be an important brick in the scientific edifice, solidifying a promising passageway to further discovery. But what this means is that scientific progress follows a well-trodden path. If you're going to pursue an unpopular area, then you may have to buck the establishment, and you may find your scientific manuscripts subject to a lot of skeptical appraisal. Not necessarily a bad thing, but probably not a situation that young, imaginative researchers would be eager to jump into.

Thirdly, scientists in universities support themselves on research grants, and these grants are given out by panels looking for the biggest bang for the buck. They want to be as certain as possible that money doled out will bring back a guaranteed return of scientific papers published in the top quality journals. So it's easy to see that pursuing a backwater area is not the surest route to success in science.

Nor, at that time, was the private sector of much help here. Big drug companies are looking for maximum return on the dollar, and pursuing epigenetic drugs would have been laughed at that time in the research planning sessions that go on in the drug companies. In the 1970s it would have been virtually impossible to predict where the field of epigenetics was headed. But you could have certainly said that wherever it was headed, it was headed there at a snail's pace.

Fourthly, you can't do scientific investigation if you lack the tools for it. As the study of genes picked up, more and better techniques and equipment for isolating and manipulating genes became available. But technologies are driven by need. Since few investigators were interested in epigenetics in 1970s and 1980s, the companies that develop the tools for laboratory investigation directed their talents toward DNA, RNA and genes, not toward the genes responding to epigenetic commands, the epigenes. It took a long time, many years, to turn around the focus of scientific investigation to reflect the intrinsic value of epigenetics.

As the interest of the scientific community in epigenetics increased during the 1990s, the companies that make the disposable kits and devices for studying this phenomenon jumped in, and what had been a vicious cycle became as virtuous cycle. A cleverly designed kit that enabled an investigator to isolate an epigene or characterize its perform-ance could mean that many experiments could be performed with greater accuracy and in a shorter time than previously was required. So the pace of publication picked up. For instance, in 1999 there were nine papers published on epigenetics in peer-reviewed journals, while in 2012 there were 4,626—about a 500-fold increase.

There's an overworked name for the introduction of a radical new model or theory into the marketplace of scientific ideas: it is referred to as a "paradigm shift." The term is frequently misused in everyday lan-guage to the point that it has become a cliché, but it is of value in under-standing how scientific discovery proceeds.

The concept was developed by the philosopher of science Thomas Kuhn, who argued that scientific revolutions occur when anomalies to a universally accepted scientific theory build to such a level that they become overwhelming.[16] Then follows an intellectual battle between the "old guard" and the "young turks," which eventually is resolved, and a new paradigm is gradually accepted. And it is always accepted, because the new paradigm is always better than the old one. By "better," we mean that it is a closer approximation of reality than the traditional theory. According to Dr. Michael Skinner, an epigeneticist at Washington State University, that is exactly what is occurring now, as the epigenetic model of inheritance becomes more widely accepted. This means that the old, dominating idea of the genomic model is no longer adequate and is gradually being replaced by the concept of an intimate relationship between the genome and the epigenome. He believes that while this change is taking place right now, it is not complete and the next few years will see a total acceptance of this concept.

How big is this paradigm shift? It is very, very big. It is not an exaggeration to say that trying to comprehend the hereditary structure of living creatures today, without taking epigenetics into account, is like trying to do physics based on pre–Einsteinian laws. That is, with Newtonian laws you can get some insights into the structure of the universe and the basic laws that govern it, but they will be incomplete. These laws, and these mathematical equations will work only under a certain range of conditions. Outside of these boundaries they will make predictions that cannot be confirmed. They will raise conundrums that cannot be resolved.

Without epigenetics we cannot understand health and disease and the laws that govern our biology. We will have an incomplete picture, one that leads into blind alleys and erroneous conclusions. Our attempts to design therapies for diseases will fail, or at best achieve only partial success.

Epigenetics Comes Out of the Closet

There are other splits within the genetics community today. Within the clan of epigenetics researchers there are actually two major groups; there may be more and there is some overlap between the two. The first body is those researchers (mainly in medical schools, drug and biotech companies) that are focusing on developing new anti-cancer drugs, based on epigenetic models. These folks are not so interested in how the patients got cancer in the first place, but rather, is the cancer epigenetically connected and if so, can you design drugs that will reverse the epigenetic changes? This is a large and very active field as we will discuss in Chapter 5. There are many other investigators looking at epigenetic drugs that target the wealth of other diseases that we will covered here, but cancer epigenetics is far ahead of the pack.

The second gaggle of investigators is mainly based in universities and research institutes and they are studying a range of epigenetic questions. Not only are they investigating the way the flow of information is epigenetically controlled in our bodies, but they are also looking at diseases other than cancer. And they are looking at environmental causes of epigenetic diseases. I will summarize in the concluding chapters some of their comments as they highlight the serious nature of epigenetic risks to our health and the quality of our environment.

We are seeing evidence of this ongoing paradigm shift throughout the scientific community. A glance at the Internet reveals dozens and dozens of products designed to make the life of epigeneticists easier and faster and more hassle-free. Learned symposia abound; there are meetings on epigenetics going on constantly all over the world. There are many journals that publish papers on epigenetics, including ones exclusively dedicated to the discipline. And research grants, the mother's milk of science that flows from the National Institutes of Health, have poured out in a flood.

However, many of the scientists that I interviewed in the preparation of this book agreed that the battle is still raging. This is because the classical way of envisioning our hereditary makeup was very straightforward: the genes are long strips of information that are read from one end to another, and then their product, the RNA, is released. This RNA is a mobile tape that transits from the cell nucleus to the cytoplasm where it hooks up with the protein-synthesizing machinery. The protein molecules are produced and their sum total constitutes the overall appearance or phenotype. Of course they must be produced at the right time and in the right place, and there are sets of signals that make this happen.

The participation of the epigenome in building the individual makes the picture much more complicated. Now we envision portions of genome that are under the control of epigenetic signals and these epigenes respond to the environment and talk back and forth to one another. The DNA is covered in many places by proteins called "histones" which respond to epigenetic triggers. The histones can come and go, depending on the messages that they are receiving. If the environment changes even slightly, this could affect the synthetic capability of these genes, and thus the overall phenotype of the individual. So the concept of epigenetics doesn't unfold naturally, and as we'll see in the coming chapters, it can be difficult to grasp, even for professionals.

All this activity must mean that we know a lot about these epigenetic molecules and what they do. While we don't know everything we would like to know, we will see in the next chapter that we are building an overall picture of what epigenes are and how they work. And we are coming to a point where we can discuss the details of their role in disease and the changes in these genes that put our survival at risk.

2

Genes: The Hardware and the Software

"What is it?"

"It's a mistake!"—Adrian Brody contemplating his latest genetically engineered monster in Splice.

The Long, Winding Molecule

DNA has become such a well-known concept in our culture today that it even forms a plot device in mainstream Hollywood films. No self-respecting science fiction film featuring creatures bubbling up in the lab would omit the requisite graphics of rotating helical DNA molecules. From *Jurassic Park* to *Spiderman* to *Contagion* to *Extraordinary Measures*, DNA plays a starring role. Clearly DNA is recognized by just about everybody as the "code of life."

The picture of graceful, spiraling molecules, whose subunits form a linear code that tells us everything about ourselves, is easy to visualize. In the years since 1953, when Watson and Crick first introduced the world to the double helix structure of DNA, the concept has become a part of the fabric of our existence. During this early period (the 1950s and 1960s), the broad mechanics of the cell and its most critical molecules, DNA, RNA and protein, were laid out.[1]

DNA was given an immense boost in the public eye during the 1990s when the sequencing of the entire DNA content of the human species was proposed. The Human Genome Project was funded through both the public and the private sectors, and received a lot of attention in the media during this period. As the work barreled along, the task became greatly simplified through new technical improvements which seemed to appear on a day to day basis. The first human genome was sequenced at a cost of around 2.7 billion dollars, much sooner and for less than had been proposed. The early sequencing work was done using primitive gene sequencer machines that worked their way down the molecules, chewing off and identifying one base at a time. Its limit was pieces of DNA with a maximum length of about 1000 bases. The technology has now advanced to a point where, using microchip devices, you can sequence a genome for around $1,000 with a slick device known as the Ion Proton Sequencer. About the size of a microwave oven and priced to sell at $149,000, it is touted as the contrivance that puts DNA sequencing into the main stream.[2]

The Human Genome Project took off in October 1990, directed by the Office of Biological and Environmental Research in the U.S. Department of Energy's Office of Science. Francis Collins directed the National Institutes of Health National Human Genome Research Institute efforts. Collins has a fine reputation as geneticist, and is well known as a folksy, guitar-playing scientist with strong Christian convictions. He is noted for his belief that science and religion are completely compatible, as he explained in *The Language of God*. The book elaborates his belief in "a consistent and profoundly satisfying harmony between 21st-century science and evangelical Christianity." Collins moved the work forward at a slow, systematic pace.

Earlier, a flamboyant and irascible iconoclast, J. Craig Venter, launched a private effort to sequence the human genome (in this case, his own) through his company, the Celera Corporation. Venter and his rival, Collins, couldn't be more different. According to *Scientific American*, "Craig Venter is the Lady Gaga of science, a drama queen, an over-the-top performance artist with a genius for self-promotion."[3] He is well-known for his voyages across the oceans of the world to collect unique genomes of marine organisms. This work has collected millions of data bits and may in time enable the development of new drugs and industrial products.

Venter has founded the J. Craig Venter Institute, and on his home page he describes himself as "one of the leading scientists of the 21st century for his numerous invaluable contributions to genomic research."

The government effort was spread among universities and research centers throughout the world. Venter, on the other hand, used $300 million of his corporation's money to race ahead, sequencing with a technique

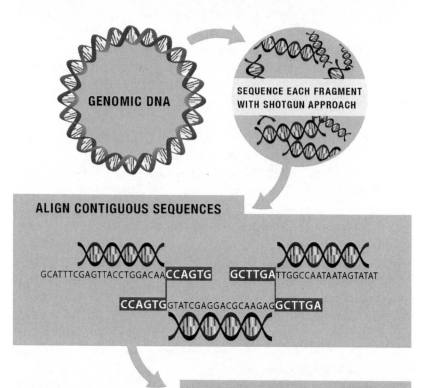

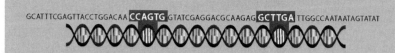

Figure 4. Whole genome shotgun sequencing. This is the basic concept for sequencing the human genome. DNA is extracted from human tissue and broken up with enzymes and other techniques into small pieces that can be handled by sequencing machines. Pieces are multiplied and introduced into sequencing machines that read off the bases one at a time. The information is stored in computers that scan for sections of overlap. This procedure was repeated millions and millions of times over the course of years of investigation by thousands of labs throughout the world. After collation and cross checking the preliminary description of the human genome was agreed upon. Drawing by Garima Naredi.

known as "shotgun sequencing," which as the name implies, involves sequencing many small pieces of DNA on a random basis. With a warehouse full of state-of-the-art sequencing machines cranking away day and night, data poured out in a deluge. At the same time, the much more methodical government program was moving ahead. Although Collins and his army of collaborators couldn't match Celera's raw speed, their information was much more structured. When a section of DNA was sequenced, you knew immediately its approximate location on one of the 23 different human chromosomes. This allowed Venter's team to match their data to the NIH information which was appearing nightly on the Internet. This meant that the random pieces could be juxtaposed into the large scale map coming from NIH. Not exactly a match made in heaven, but the two strategies complemented one another, and put the sequencing project on steroids.

Americans love a competition, but the race became nasty as the publicly and privately funded efforts went up cheek to jowl against one another. There was considerable sniping between the two sides, causing unwanted attention in the media. By 2000 this disagreement was a major embarrassment to the Democratic administration. To resolve the animosity, President Bill Clinton, in Solomonic fashion, declared the genome sequenced and chopped the genome baby in half, presenting a portion to Collins, the head of the government funded project, and the other half to Venter, the head of the private effort.[4] However, the genome was still a premature baby, and represented only a rough map, with many portions yet to be filled in. It would not be until 2003 that a complete sequence would be available.

In the years since, the Human Genome Project has proven to be immensely successful as a technical triumph (it has been compared to the NASA space exploration effort). Thousands of species, from viruses to jellyfish to frogs to dogs and cats and people, have enjoyed the sequencing of their genomes. In many instances, thousands of members of a given species have been sequenced, so we know the amount of variation from individual to individual. There has been an outpouring of discoveries resulting from these projects, triumphs in evolutionary biology, ecology, forensics and epidemiology. Some of the more exotic choices include the puffer fish, the elephant, the sea urchin, the lamprey, and the Tasmanian devil.

However, it did not produce the bounty of new treatments for diseases that its supporters had promised. Even today there are very few new drugs or tests for diseases that can be directly attributed to the human genome project. This proved to be somewhat of an embarrassment in an era of cost-cutting and demands from congress to justify every expenditure in terms of immediate profit.[5]

It turns out that the diseases that are the main causes of death and disability have an extremely complex basis. When the genome was searched for genes that contribute to cardiovascular diseases, many were identified, but each proved to be a small contributor to the condition, and some may have been statistical aberrations.[6] And unfortunately, they were not of much value in predicting individuals that would fall victim to stroke or heart attack. In fact, in a 2010 interview, Craig Venter said, "We have, in truth, learned nothing from the genome other than probabilities. How does a 1 or 3 percent increased risk for something translate into the clinic? It is useless information."[7]

The Epigenome Rises

Why didn't the human genome project lead to new cures for disease? If you knew the identification and location of every one of the 3 billion or so bases in the genome, wouldn't that provide all the information that you needed? Wouldn't this enable you to link diseases to the genome, and wouldn't this allow you to treat them successfully?

The answer is a resounding no. In the first place, the information encoded in the genome is not self-explanatory. This groaning volume of genetic code was largely written in a foreign language. There had to be a vast array of controller genes and other regulatory features that could not be pinpointed at that time. It would require years of research to sort out these elements and understand how they relate to one another.

And bear in mind that in the 1990s, the focus was on the genome, not the epigenome. That means that the sequencing technology was aimed entirely at the DNA code, and the epigenome was pretty much ignored. So this map of countless adenines, guanines, thymines and cytosines running off into infinity didn't tell the whole story; maybe in order to relate a coherent vision you needed additional information that hadn't been allowed in the original program.

Because of this lag in the focus of genetic research, the "epigenome" is today not as well understood as the genome, but it is now receiving a great deal of attention. This is because the sequencing of the human and many other genomes failed to explain the nature of the forces that control how genes are activated and inactivated, which is precisely where the epigenomics story comes in.[8]

Think of the genome as the hardware, the information that's permanent. Like the structures that make up a computer, the DNA is hard-wired, built into the organism. This doesn't mean that it never changes, but by and large, it's going to be a pretty rare event. But if you have the hardware, then there must be signals, signposts that tell the hardware how to respond. So certain arrangements of bases along the DNA identify triggers that would activate or inactivate the genes coded in the DNA.

This is where the software comes in. The structures of the DNA bases can be modified chemically by addition of small molecules to the original framework. One of the best studied of these is methylation sites, stretches of DNA where a lot of cytosines are located. When methyl groups (a carbon atom and three hydrogens) attach to these cytosines, they form a block in the long, spiraling helix that prevents the genes from being read (or "expressed") and making whatever proteins they are coded to produce. Conversely, if you remove the methyl groups, the signaling genes allow the reading of the gene to proceed. So the epigenetic sites are on/off switches that regulate the "structural" genes that make all the proteins that constitute the "phenotype," the overall appearance and performance of the individual.

There are a number of other groups of chemical modifiers that attach to the DNA and affect its behavior. Histones are proteins that interact with DNA (often through methylation sites). They can form big mufflers, interacting with the DNA so whole stretches of chromosomes are shut off, and fail to produce any signals for protein production. Since the histones are large molecules, they have a lot of places where chemical reactions can change them slightly. These changes affect their ability to control the expression of genes to which they are connected. These different reactions yield a menu of slightly altered molecules, sort

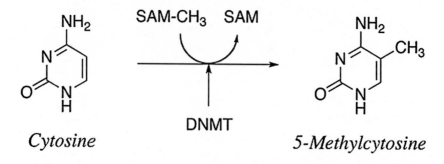

Figure 5. DNA methylation. This is the classic chemical step, by which a tag is placed on the cytosine molecules in the DNA which allows it to act as a marker, regulating the reading of genes in the DNA. Only certain cytosines in the DNA are selected to take part in this reaction.

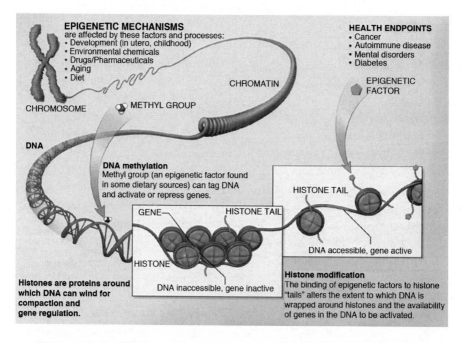

Figure 6. Role of Histones in Epigenetic Control. Histones are proteins which complex with the DNA in order to drive gene regulation. Histone modification occurs when the binding of epigenetic factors to histone "tails" alters the binding of the DNA to the histones, allowing specific genes to be activated. Courtesy National Human Genome Research Institute.

of like the Baskin-Robbins ice cream flavors (the same basic ingredients, with minor modifications), although their technical names aren't quite so appetizing: acetylation, methylation, phosphorylation, and so forth. Some of these modifications to the histones will cause them to make genes work harder; some will cause them to dampen the genes' output.[9]

The histones are managed by three different groups of protein known as "readers," "writers" and "erasers." The first group, the epigenetic "writer" proteins, alter histones by adding an acetyl group. This modification blocks the ability of the histone to bind DNA, opening it up and allowing its messages to be read. On the other hand the "eraser" proteins remove the acetyl group from the histones restoring the interaction between the histone and DNA, leaving the DNA once again in a closed conformation. The result: no message read. Finally, the epigenetic "readers" don't alter the histones but rather detect the acetyl group within the histones.

Yet another form of epigenetic control resides in what are known as "microRNAs." It has been recognized for 50 years or more that an intermediate molecule in the cell, RNA, carries information from the nucleus to the cytoplasm of the cell, where dedicated machinery translates the RNA into protein. These RNAs are read off one strand of the DNA, and since they carry a message, they are known as messenger RNA. On the other hand, the microRNAs are epigenetically controlled, very small RNA molecules, that complex with the messenger RNAs and prevent their functioning. They don't code for proteins, as the messenger RNA does. Often these microRNAs are arrayed in groups, so they form complexes that control many genes. They can act as "dimmer switches" on the messengers, so they make less protein.

The rule that emerges is that epigenetic control is based on molecular locks and keys, molecules that complex with informational molecules and shut off their function. This is a familiar pattern in biology, in which organisms are a great network of on/off switches all talking back and forth, constantly responding to the environmental changes going on around them. There's even a branch of the life sciences, systems biology, that specializes in the study of interactive networks in living creatures.

So the epigenetic systems are set up to respond, at the appropriate time, to chemical signals that appear at just the right moment in the development of the embryo. When it's all set up and waiting, the chemical signal comes in from another gene, it turns on the epigenes and everything moves smoothly ahead. Unless it doesn't. That is, if a false message comes in from the outside, that turns on the epigenetic switches at the wrong moment, too early or too late, or forces too much or too little gene product.

So we can state that epigenetic mechanisms can affect the overall appearance (the phenotype) without changes to the basic DNA code. But there's more: epigenetic changes can be reversed, whereas DNA changes are by and large permanent. The other important feature is that epigenetic changes can be passed on to subsequent generations. This means that master switches could be shut on or off in a semi-permanent state, a very different property from the hardwired DNA. We still haven't talked about how these switches are activated and inactivated, and this question will bring us to the heart of the concept of epigenetics.

Control Freak

Because DNA is a long linear molecule, it's easy to imagine the information content of our DNA as a line of type on a printed page, albeit a very long line, since the entire human hereditary message is around three billion bases. To give you some comparison, this book is about a half million letters long, so it would take 1.5 thousand books such as this one to match the information content of one human genome. A big book indeed. In fact in 2012 a group of scientists at the University of Leicester decided to print out a complete hard copy version of the human genome.[10] It ran to 130 volumes, with each page printed on both sides in 4-point font, with precisely 43,000 characters per page. The X chromosome alone took up seven volumes, while the Y chromosome (which determines maleness and not much else) occupies one. The exercise cost a little less than £4,000 (about $6,000).

In the early days of molecular biology, genes were discovered in bacteria that controlled other genes. Bacteria live in a constantly changing environment; if you're a bacterium, one minute you're safe and sound in the intestine, the next you're on your way down the Mississippi River. Thus it's not surprising that many of these controller genes responded

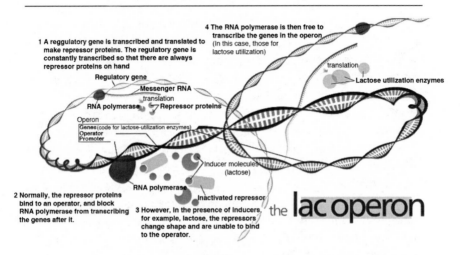

Figure 7. The operon. The operon is the classic model of gene regulation, developed from studies on bacteria and bacterial virus during the 1950s and '60s. It proposes a simple and elegant model of how the flow of genetic information is controlled in lower forms, but its relevance is limited in higher organisms.

to signals such as the availability of food in the environment. If a particular indigestible sugar were present, the controller genes would respond by activating a gene that made an enzyme that could break down the sugar so that the bacterial cell could gobble it up.

The entire unit is known as the "Operon," and it was discovered over 50 years ago. It consists of a gene called a promoter, followed by a second gene, the operator, and then followed by a group of structural genes, whose job is to make proteins. Ordinarily, all the genes are turned off (why waste your energy making something that you cannot use?) because a molecule called a repressor is built to sit on the operator gene and nothing moves ahead. But when a sugar (lactose) is present, it kicks the repressor molecule off the operator. Now the promoter is freed up, and the gene starts cranking. And they produce the protein enzymes that attack the sugar. The lactose is broken down to a form that the bacterial cell can use for its nutritional needs (see Figure 7). This is such a neat mechanism that it captured the imagination of scientists all over the world. Eventually its discovers, Francois Jacob, Jacque Monod and André Lwoff, would win the Nobel prize.[11]

Jacob is the only living member of the trio.[12] Originally trained as a physician, he fought so bravely during World War II that he was awarded the *croix de guerre*, France's highest decoration for valor. Now in his 90s, he recently explained how he came upon such an amazing piece of science: "Our breakthrough was the result of 'night science': a stumbling, wandering exploration of the natural world that relies on intuition as much as it does on the cold, orderly logic of 'day science'. In today's vastly expanded scientific enterprise, obsessed with impact factors and competition, we will need much more night science to unveil the many mysteries that remain about the workings of organisms."

In the months and years following the revelations of the operon model, molecular biologists assumed that higher organisms used a similar, perhaps more intricate approach, but more or less the same idea with more bells and whistles. But much effort to uncover "operons" in mammals ended in failure. Only in recent years have rare examples of operon-like complexes been observed in higher organisms, including mammals.[13]

Epigenetics: All About Control

With the rise of the epigenetics paradigm, we see that the earlier notions concerning how the information flow was controlled were hopelessly inadequate, because they didn't recognize modulation through epigenetic signals. It turned out that all higher organisms possessed DNA decorated with proteins, the histones, as we discussed previously. These histones bind to the DNA and their pattern of binding is part of the epigenetic modulation of gene expression. In the many stages that cells go through in the course of reproduction, the histones interact with the DNA to turn genes on and off at the appropriate times.

This means that almost all the genes are turned off in the sperm and egg cells. Following fertilization an activation process occurs, and the fertilized egg divides over and over again. So these complex networks begin to spark and flash, and a busy conversation begins. The chatter is incessant, but perfectly timed and coordinated as the embryo proceeds in its development. These events must occur at the precisely correct moments. If not, the results could be anywhere from trivial or barely detectable all the way to catastrophic. The possible damage could include birth defects, mental retardation and late onset diseases such as Alzheimer's and Parkinson's. This is why the concept of epigenetic control is so critical to human health—because we are learning that these control mechanisms are extremely fragile. Let's see exactly how and why the genes are so delicate, and what forces, natural or manmade, may disrupt them.

3

Mutations and Epimutations

Hiroshima, Mon Amour

For Keijiro Matsushima and his 16-year-old classmates in the city of Hiroshima, August 6, 1945, started as an ordinary day, a beautiful crystalline blue sky bathing the city in morning light. At 8:15 he was just starting to focus on his calculus lessons when he looked out of the school room window and saw a couple of American B29 bombers overhead. He didn't worry much; Hiroshima had never been bombed and he assumed they were there for surveillance. Then in an instant everything disappeared in a tremendous explosion.

"There was a very strong flash and a heat wave," he related in a recent interview. "The whole world turned into something orange. I felt like I was thrown into an oven for a moment."[1]

In those seconds, up to 80,000 lives were extinguished as the city was transformed into a raging inferno. In the days following the blast, Matsushima, who is alive today, came to learn that a new weapon, the atomic bomb, had devastated his city and the neighboring Japanese city of Nagasaki. He was fortunate to have not been seriously injured and was able to escape from Hiroshima and join his mother who was living outside of the city. He suffered radiation sickness and subsequently recovered.

Matsushima had no way of knowing at the time, but he and the other survivors of the atomic bomb blasts would be followed and their health status assessed for years afterward by the Atomic Bomb Casualty Commission, which later became the Radiation Effects Research Foundation. Sixty-nine years later, this agency is still in operation, and is charged with considering the effects of radiation on the health of the survivors, their children and their grandchildren.

Why is this work so important? Couldn't we gain the same information by studying lab animals and tissue culture cells? The answer to this question is a resounding no. This is because despite similarities, humans are different from lab animals. We live much longer, and so we must have ways of maintaining the stability of our genomes over a period of many decades; mice and rats live about two years, so they wouldn't need the same level of protection. The bomb survivors represent a large number of individuals, and the amount of radiation they received is accurately known. Since there are two biological consequences which we are investigating, we need to have accurate numbers for cancers and numbers of mutations caused by a unit of radiation.

It is not enough to simply provide a vague statement, such as "radiation caused some mutations in the DNA that can be passed on to subsequent generations and radiation causes some cancers." If the government is to establish tolerable doses of radiation from medical and industrial sources it needs to have as accurate a number as possible. These are the data that allow agencies such as the EPA to establish exposure guidelines to be used in industry and medicine.

The Genome: Stable as a Rock

In putting together our story of the genome versus the epigenome, we have seen that the genome, or the genetic hardware, is quite stable. The base pairs in the DNA don't change often, and it's a good thing they don't. If they did, plant and animal species wouldn't have any permanence. We know this isn't true, since many creatures have been around for millions and millions of years. For instance, sharks, ferns and horseshoe crabs can be found in ancient fossil records, virtually unchanged. Cockroach-like fossils from the Carboniferous period between 354 and 295 million years ago are very much like their nasty modern cousins that you may encounter in your kitchen when you come in during the middle of the night and turn on the lights.

In fact, some scientists have suggested that DNA is the most stable thing in the universe. It is hard to imagine anything more enduring. "Our love will last forever," goes the romantic ballad, yet it is over in the twinkling of an eye. Our civilizations, our architecture, our human institutions all fade away in the course of the centuries. In 300 million years, mountains wash down to the sea, the stars change their courses, whole planetary systems are transformed. Yet DNA remains.[2] One of the many epigeneticists that I interviewed for this book, John McCarrey at the University of Texas at San Antonio, explains it this way: "In the case of the genome, we are exposed to thousands of potentially mutagenic effects per cell per day. However, the vast majority of those do NOT cause a permanent mutation in our DNA because we have DNA repair mechanisms that recognize the initial effect (DNA damage) and correct (repair) the problem to restore and maintain the original DNA sequence."

When geneticists were making their first forays into the study of heredity a century ago, they focused on plants and animals that are cheap to raise and easy to keep, like fruit flies. They observed that there were discrete "factors" that yielded alternate patterns or "phenotypes." When flies with different phenotypes were crossed with one another, the progeny showed these phenotypes in different predictable ratios. From these observations they could draw conclusions about the factors (or "genotypes") that determined the outcome of the offspring.

But there was a real problem. If you looked at these little beasties, they all looked pretty much the same, so you didn't have much to work with. Virtually all the fruit flies had red eyes, and the investigators were very lucky to discover a fly with white eyes. These few rare "sports" or variants were gradually accumulated, but locating these needles in haystacks was a very slow and laborious process. So work moved at an agonizingly sluggish pace. But by the 1920s a number of people working in genetics realized that the incidence of mutation could be ramped up many times by exposing the parent plant or animal to X-rays. If you had a means of detecting these newly minted critters, you could produce a whole collection of new possibilities, enough to keep you busy for years. One of these scientists was H. J. Muller, who won the Nobel Prize for demonstrating that X-rays caused mutations in fruit flies.

Muller was a colorful figure himself, who in terms of his audacity could certainly stand up to any of his modern day counterparts. Disenchanted with the misery of the Depression-era United States, he left for Europe shortly after he published some of his most important scientific work. Between 1933 and 1936 he worked in the Soviet Union, where he was quite productive until the excesses of Stalinist Russia became too much for him to bear. Forced to leave, he rambled about Europe for some time. He is said to have fought in the Spanish Civil War and eventually made it back to the United States.[3]

Muller was passionate and outspoken in his leftwing political philosophy. These "youthful indiscretions" made his life difficult in the post–World War II era, when congressional subcommittees were looking for communists under every bed. He scrambled to find a job at a time when intellectuals who had defected to the Soviet Union were highly suspect. Fortunately for Muller, the Chancellor at Indiana University was familiar with his accomplishments, and offered him a job in 1945. He won the Nobel Prize in 1946, which gave him the stature to push for the responsible management of X-rays and other forms of radiation.[4] As one of the world's foremost experts on the dangers of radiation, he helped raise concerns over nuclear fallout, which led to the nuclear test ban treaty in 1962.

Muller's life was summarized for me one day when I was in graduate school by Lawrence Sandler, one of my mentors. "Muller was an incredible thinker," he related to me. "Every significant concept in genetics, he conceived of it first."[5]

Mutations and Cancer

Today with our intimate knowledge of the human genome, we are a world away from Muller's understanding of the nature of mutations and the role of radiation in their origins. One of the major contributors to these insights has been the ongoing studies on the atom bomb survivors. This work has established that the survivors had higher rates of cancer, especially leukemia. Powerful blasts of electromagnetic energy, including x-rays, damage genes by knocking atoms off the DNA molecules and causing breaks and other lesions. And this damage can bend normal body cells to become tumor cells. For this reason, there is much effort to guard patients from being exposed to unnecessary doses of X-rays. Over the years these efforts have been largely successful, due to improvements in the technology. Medical X-ray machines are infinitely better engineered today, so their beams are focused, rather than spraying the radiation all over the place. Thus only the target area is exposed,

41

resulting in much lower overall doses to patients. In addition, the sensitivity of X-ray film has been tremendously improved over the years and is gradually being abandoned entirely in favor of digital technology, which delivers only one fifth the dose of the best film imaging.

Despite their hazards to humans and other living creatures, X-rays and other forms of ionizing radiation were found to be extremely useful in cancer research, both in diagnosis and treatment. Much of what is known about oncology in humans has come from these studies.

In the second half of the 20th century chemicals were discovered that could also produce mutations and cancers in experimental animals. These substances are known as alkylating agents, and they were the original basis of World War I's nerve gas. They were referred to as mustard gases, and they were so deadly that they haven't been used since for military purposes. But they turned out to be a two-edged sword, serving as the basis of modern chemotherapy for cancer treatment. The alkylating agents kill dividing cells, and rapidly dividing cancer cells can be targeted in this fashion.

The Epigenome: Not So Stable

If the genome is so stable, and rarely changes, what about the epigenome? We've already spoken of the unusual properties of the epigenome, the stretches of DNA, the genes, that are under control of the sections of DNA that respond to epigenetic signals. These sections have been given a name—one of these regions, for example, is referred to as "CpG Islands" but your travel agent won't be able book a trip for you to visit them. Think of them as clusters of cytosines alternating with guanines, forming a milepost along the DNA. When these CpG islands and other shorter regions are worked over by the methylation reaction, they block the reading of the genes to which they are adjacent. So this means they won't produce the messenger RNA, and no protein will be synthesized. This could prove devastating to the host, depending on the gene's function.

It turns out that epigenomic sites ARE subject to changes that can have profound effects on the individual's phenotype, and we will see that this dampening or shutting off of the flow of information can occur with great frequency under the right conditions. So evidence is piling up that epigenomic changes are much more frequent than changes in the DNA base pair sequences. When living systems are exposed to radiation, they can cause damage directly to the DNA (genomic mutations) or disrupt the methylation of the CpG islands or shorter stretches that are just two bases long, the CpG dinucleotides, and destroy effective control of gene expression (epigenomic mutations). So the two types of changes are intertwined.

John McCarrey explained it this way: "In all likelihood the epigenome is labile and highly sensitive. We get tens of thousands of potential mutagenic hits to the DNA per day per cell and we repair the vast majority of these. We have a nice mechanism to protect the genome, but we don't have a mechanism to protect the epigenome. It is sitting out there exposed without protection, as far as we know. So we must be encountering these effects all the time."

McCarrey goes on to say that the majority of epimutations will not be passed on to subsequent generations, because most (but apparently not all) are eliminated in the process of egg and sperm formation. But you can readily appreciate that epimutations could cause a great deal of mischief to the individual in which they occur. In particular organs, they could cause malignant transformations, as well as many other highly undesirable changes.

"In contrast, we have no such immediate repair mechanism that can recognize or repair environmentally induced damage to the epigenome. So it is likely we maintain epigenetic defects (epimutations) in cells that encounter these disruptions. The one place where such defects can potentially be corrected is in the germ line (sperm in males and eggs/oocytes in females). As a normal facet of development of the germ line in each sex, inherited epigenetic programming is erased and reset. So, in theory, this should erase correct OR incorrect programming (including epimutations) and only correct programming should be restored when the epigenome is reset in germ cells. We have examples where this sort of 'germline correction' clearly does occur. However, we also have examples where this does not seem to occur, though we still don't understand why or how certain epimutations appear to escape the normal epigenetic reprogramming process in the germ line."

The Toxic Soup du Jour

The alkylating agents were some of the early contributors to the industrial-medical chemical industry. Over the years the number of chemicals introduced into our environment has skyrocketed to around 80,000, but this is only a guess, since we really don't have a solid accounting.[6] They have been invented for medical, dietary, artistic and industrial purposes, and many are essential to our modern way of life. Some have been tested in the laboratory to see whether they cause tumors in experimental animals, but this is not a foolproof approach, and in any case the numbers that have been looked at are infinitesimal compared to the thousands of chemicals that douse our civilization.

It is most ironic that the same agents that are used to treat and kill cancer cells can also cause new cancers. In fact, CT scans, which deliver a lot of radiation, may be responsible for as much as 1.5 to 2 percent of all cancers. Since the probability of having cancer during your lifetime is around one in four or 25 percent, this doesn't raise your risk much on an individual level, but the total numbers of cancer is quite substantial. But these estimates are subject to many caveats and it will be some time before really firm, reliable numbers associated with these risk factors are possible.[7] Especially the possibility of a threshold effect, discussed later on in this chapter.

Theories concerning the origins of cancer focused on the genome; they suggested that some agent in the environment or some unknown event altered the base pair code of the DNA, causing mutations that affected one or more of the many genes known to control normal growth. With the rapid sequencing technologies that have seen so much improvement in recent years, there are at least 1500 genes related to cancer that have been discovered. A fairly straightforward theory of cancer based on these observations tells us that mutations in different members of this collection caused the genes to function inappropriately, and the cells started down the long road to malignancy. After enough mutations accumulated, the cell became destabilized and moved into a self-perpetuating cycle of disarray. This concept has received a lot of support as tumor cell genes have been sequenced and many DNA-based mutations have been identified.

But the picture has turned out to be a lot more complicated. So

44

while this theory was popular for years, it always had its detractors, spoil-sports who showed up to rain on the parade. One of the major failings of the genome mutation theory was that as more and more chemicals were classified as carcinogens or cancer causing substances, it became clear that many were not mutation-causing in the classical sense, as are the alkylating agents and X-rays. For instance, inflammation is blamed for causing many types of cancer, and it is certainly not a mutation-causing agent. Likewise, lousy diet and poor lifestyle habits (such as sitting on your rear in front of a computer all day) are correlated with elevated cancer rates, and they couldn't possibly be considered classical DNA mutagens. Hormones and hormone-like compounds are another class of risk factors, and they do not cause base pair changes in the DNA.

Who Did It? Tracking Down the Malefactor

If you're a good murder mystery wonk, you can probably see where we're headed. We've seen that the qualities of the genome make it clear that classical mutations alone cannot explain all the features of cancer cells. Not only do a lot of chemicals not thought to be mutagenic in the classical sense cause cancers, there are documented cases of cancers spontaneously resolving back to a state of normalcy.

But how can this be? There are two terrible types of cancer, melanoma (a really nasty skin cancer) and neuroblastoma (a cancer of the neurons, one of the classes of brain cells) that sometimes disappear spontaneously.[8] This hardly makes sense if cancer is due to a mutation-like change, since we would expect this to be a one-way affair. That is, the DNA is quite stable, and when it rarely changes, it doesn't change back. But if we take into account the epigenome, then the picture becomes a lot more complicated, but a lot closer to reality. The theory that is now emerging is that cancer is the result of alteration in the genome and the epigenome, and these changes play back and forth upon one another.

It turns out that there is now a lot of new research that ties epigenomic changes to cancer causation, and this is raising serious concerns over uncontrolled and unregulated exposure to chemicals that interact

45

with the epigenome. But unfortunately this is only a part of the story. There are many other diseases that have seen rapid increases in their incidence, and circumstantial evidence suggested an epigenetic cause. Now the evidence is much stronger, and many scientists feel that it is no longer "circumstantial."

Radiation Increases Cancer Rates, Both Genomic and Epigenomic

This brings us back to the question that was posed by the studies of the Japanese atomic bomb victims with which we began this story. What have 64 years of investigation told us about the effects of radiation on the human genome?

After some years of study it was determined that cancer rates among the survivors were somewhat elevated, but many investigations, conducted in a variety of ways, have never shown a statistically significant increase in the rates of mutations among the children or grandchildren of the survivors who were exposed to radiation from the blasts. As the years have passed the studies have become more and more sophisticated, examining changes in the DNA codes, breaks in chromosomes, a possible increase in inherited diseases among children of survivors, and some indirect methods of getting at changes in the DNA. All of these studies came up negative. This seems contradictory, because we know that radiation causes mutation in a wide range of lab animals and plants.

There can be no doubt that humans are sensitive to radiation effects, since our biology is so similar to other mammals. This makes it difficult to understand why the effects observed are not more dramatic. There are two possible explanations. The first is that even among those survivors that received the highest doses of radiation, the amounts were too low to produce a measurable effect. The second, and much more interesting, is that there is a threshold, a level below which radiation will not produce mutations because the organism can repair small amounts of damage, as shown in Figure 8. This is still a highly controversial and politically charged issue, because all the protective standards that have been established over the years by regulatory bodies such

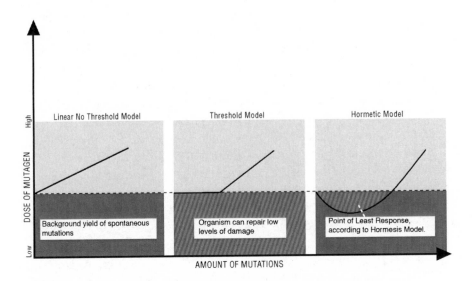

Figure 8. Mutations and Epimutations. Graph shows three possible responses of the hereditary material to radiation, chemicals or other mutagenic agents. The classic, conventional assumption is that the more of mutagen applied to the genetic material, the more damage (linear response). The starting point represents the base line "spontaneous" mutation frequency. Other models propose that at very low doses there is no effect, because minor damage can be cleaned up by the cell's repair mechanisms (threshold; second graph). A third possibility is known as hormesis. In this case, the chemical produces what is known as a *biphasic dose–response* relationship, exerting an opposite effect dependent on the dose. There is evidence that this response occurs in the case of epimutagens, a proposal that has attracted interest in the field of carcinogenesis. Drawing by Garima Naredi.

as the EPA have assumed there is no threshold. But we know that all organisms have systems that repair damage to their DNA, and these systems are well-known and extensively investigated in humans. They consist of a family of enzymes that set to work on damaged DNA, and attempt to put it back in order.

Why is this so important, and why is it politically sensitive? Because if small amounts of damage can be repaired by our natural defenses, then all the acceptable levels that have been in place for years would have to be reevaluated. This would include devices such as dental and medical X-ray machines, as well as radiation exposure levels to workers in industries that use radiation and radioisotopes. It would also apply to warnings concerning radon levels in houses and other environmental exposures. It could well mean that our government has spent huge amounts of money protecting people from an exaggerated threat. This would no doubt prove to be highly embarrassing to regulatory agencies that have set "no threshold" standards in place for decades.

It could also mean that the use of radioactivity for industrial purposes, such as nuclear power plants, may need to be reevaluated. If there is a threshold, then estimates of the damage from the Chernobyl accident may be too high. In the years following the accident, many estimates were made of the number of excess deaths from cancer, and the number vary wildly, from a 27,000 to over 250,000, depending on the assumptions that are made.[9] Recent investigations[10] have not been able to demonstrate an increase in cancer rates among a Finnish population exposed to low levels of radiation in the first decade after the accident. These articles point out how difficult it is to collect meaningful data and draw scientifically valid conclusions from environmental exposure to radiation. A recent paper concludes, "Our findings indicate limited data and statistical flaws. Other confounding factors, make interpretation of the results from the published literature difficult. We have learned little of the consequences of radiation exposure at Chernobyl except for its effects on thyroid cancer incidence."[11]

A lower effect of radiation on cancer rates would provide an argument for the nuclear power industry to push construction of more power plants, even in the face of accidents such as the recent 2012 Fukushima disaster. There are of course many other concerns, such as the cost of nuclear power, and the risks of acute exposure to high levels of radiation which are known to be hazardous.

Almost all of the studies that we have so far mentioned were performed prior to the "epigenetics revolution." Recent studies with lab animals have demonstrated that radiation can induce damage to epigenomic and genomic structures, so it is understandable why the atomic bomb survivors showed increases in rates of leukemia. The genetic studies looked for DNA mutations, and were not designed to detect epigenetic alterations. At this point it is probably too late to gather such information. There are other ongoing studies of radiation workers and other groups of individuals who accidentally received high levels of radiation and these may help to answer these very critical questions.[12]

Hiroshima Redux

Years of research and painstaking investigation are coming together to paint a picture of our genetic endowment, the genome based on DNA that is quite stable, and even when abused, repairs itself. But now we know that this is only part of the story; the other component is the epigenome, and we are learning that it is much more fragile and unstable. The regions of the genome that are subject to epigenetic regulation constitute this epigenome and they can be affected by many different environmental insults. This means that these two intertwined systems form a constantly shifting complex, and we cannot understand how genes are controlled without a grasp of how this complex interacts. While our current understanding is not clear in all its details, it is sufficient to consider the risks, hazards and how to mitigate them.

I started this discussion of the stability of the genome and epigenome with a mention of Keijiro Matsushima, one of the victims of the only wartime use of atomic weapons in history. According to the CNN interview, the recent tsunami in Japan brought back painful memories for him. "It's like the third atomic bomb attack on Japan," he stated, "but this time, we made it ourselves."

Matsushima has spent his life calling attention to the horrors of that terrible day so long ago, in the hopes that the world will not forget. In the years to come we will see whether the damage inflicted by these weapons was a warning of much worse threats to come.

4

Epigenetics:
What Makes It Unique?

The View from Thirty Thousand Feet

A stylized picture of the genome is a display of billions of DNA bases, strung out endlessly in linear arrays, like a highway, a railroad map, or a complex of highways. This is not what our genome really looks like, since it must be wound up and spooled and compressed so as to fit into the nucleus of a cell. This means there are three-dimensional structures that allow a yard or so of DNA to be crammed into such a tiny space. But let's pretend for the time being that the DNA could be spread out flat so we can appreciate the individual features along the road map.

What we see is that a lot of the DNA doesn't make proteins; in fact, this was long thought of as "junk," but these sections are now known to run herd on the genes that produce proteins, helping to regulate them and do their functions at the appropriate time and place. It's been shown only recently that there are thousands of controlling genes packed away in this so-called junk which really isn't junk at all. There's also lots of repeating sequences that are found at the ends and various points along the chromosomes. Interspersed between these regions are coding genes, and these genes have other genes in front of them called promoters that signal protein synthesis to proceed. But about half the genes also have the so-called CpG islands in front of them. As we saw in the last chapter, these are important for epigenetic control, and when these regions are blocked, the genes can't make their proteins. This is the part of the genome that we call the "epigenome," because we use non–DNA base pair instructions to turn these sequences on and off.

There are also histones that form tight bundles that are wrapped around the DNA. The precise arrangement of the DNA and histones is not so well understood. A third category is the microRNAs, that modulate gene activity, also epigenetically controlled. This all sounds pretty obtuse, and if you were able to look at a wiring diagram of the genome and epigenome (which is not possible today because it hasn't been figured out yet), it would be an indecipherable mess.

But if you were to look at the wiring blueprints for a modern skyscraper, they would appear pretty overwhelming, yet such instructions are used by builders all over the world. And the folks that do this are not rocket scientists. There are layers of complexity in both the case of a human construct or the cells that we have considered. In fact, the complexity of a single cell in our bodies is more at the level of a city than a single building; it would be wonderful if we understood it completely, but we don't need that level of detail to understand the workings of the genome and the epigenome.

The bottom line is that the two systems coexist within the cell; they interact with one another and both are vital for normal functioning of living creatures. But we're finding that the epigenome is much more plastic and flexible, and it can respond in unanticipated ways to environmental effects.

So What's the Difference?

Let's all admit that biology is complicated (how many cures for cancer were announced this week?). Further, let's accept the model that there are two systems at play here, and that they're intertwined and overlapping. And let's note that although we don't know everything about genomics and epigenomics, we do know a lot, and new information is emerging on a daily basis.

But why does it matter? Aside from the intrinsic intellectual charm of the idea, what is it about an understanding of epigenetics that is really a game changer? Don't these observations simply mean that heredity is very complicated? Didn't we already know that? Will an understanding of epigenetics have an impact on our day to day lives? Will it affect political and social discourse?

I would answer all of the above in the affirmative.

I would argue that the concept of the epigenome is a revolutionary, game changing concept. Understanding its place in modern biology and how it is imperiled stacks right up there with the major challenges to our civilization. Resolving this menace to our survival will occupy our energies and resources for years to come. Why?

The (Limited) Staying Power of Epigenetics

We've seen that a hallmark of the epigenome is its instability. This means that although it determines functions that are essential for survival, there are natural and artificial forces that can change the expression of the epigenome, with shattering consequences. But there's something we have touched on only peripherally, and that's the fact that once the changes take place, they can be retained in cells descended from the epigenetically affected cells, and there is evidence that in some cases these changes can be passed through the generations.

Until recently, it has been assumed that if genes were epigenetically modified, these changes would be wiped clean in every generation. That is, when the egg and sperm were formed that would come together to produce the next generation, any epigenetic modifications to the single sequences or to the CpG islands or other epigenetic signals along the road map would be erased and a brand new, clean program would be set up. This was what had been observed for some of the major changes that take place in the chromosomes, as they prepare for their transition to the next cycle of reproduction. But now evidence is building that not only can factors such as stress, nutritional deprivation, drugs and neuronal stimulation produce epigenetic changes in humans and experimental animals, but these changes can be transgenerational, meaning that they can be established in one generation and transmitted to the offspring. This does not apply to all signals, but there is evidence accumulating that it does affect a number of epigenetically determined traits.

These are such striking claims that they deserve some explanation and supporting evidence. Because what I am arguing is that the major diseases that plague the human race can be affected by factors such as stress that force epigenetic changes in cells, causing them to misperform.

Furthermore, other types of environmental damage can cause permanent epigenetic damage that could be perpetuated for generations.

This does not mean that epigenetic changes are solely responsible for these diseases. All these conditions are complex, and I will stress over and over again that the picture that is emerging is one in which the genome, the epigenome and the environment all come together to produce the particular disease.

Diseases, Revealed and Uncovered?

I'm sticking with a broad picture, in keeping with the goal of this chapter. When I argue concerning the role that epigenetics plays in individual diseases, we'll talk about the fine points.

There are a number of ways that we try to understand a disease process and the possible effective therapies. We can use tissue culture, in which cells are cultivated in liquid media. We can use small animals, usually mice and rats. We can use primates, monkeys or even great apes, such as chimpanzees. We can study populations of humans that were exposed to the conditions that we wish to understand; we can select on the basis of age, sex or other criteria and analyze the results statistically. Or we can set up clinical trials, in which volunteers with a particular disease are tested for their response to a drug or therapy. The evaluation of hazardous substances, causation of diseases and the various therapies is usually a combination of these approaches.

All of these methods have their advantages and disadvantages, so we would want to combine as many of these strategies as possible. If the results collected from different lines of evidence are in agreement this will give us more confidence in our search for the "smoking gun."

Tissue culture cells are grown in plastic flasks, and they may stick to the surface and form layers, or they may lack the ability to grab on to the flask surface, and grow as a suspension. They're maintained in incubators at body temperature, and they do quite well. They have the advantage that you can douse them with chemicals that cause epigenetic changes ("epigenetic mutagens"), you can analyze both normal cells and cancerous cells, you can check the DNA for genomic and epigenomic changes and you can repeat the experiment as many times as you wish.[1]

Other investigators in other labs can obtain cells from your laboratory and duplicate your work under the precise same conditions. The cells can be frozen and brought back to life; in short, it's a system over which the investigator has complete control. The disadvantages are that these cells are a far cry from an actual patient or subject, and there are many limitations: cells don't have livers, kidneys or other organs so they can't break down and metabolize toxins or drugs the way a real animal can. Moreover, cells cultivated for extended periods in culture may undergo transformational changes that alter their behavior in ways that are unpredictable.

Animal models are better, although they lack the tight control that cell culture offers. Almost all of the animal experimentation that goes on today is performed with rodents, since larger animals are very expensive for reasons that we will get into in a minute. Rats and mice are real animals and they have many features that cells in culture lack. But their life spans are short, and their metabolism is very different in myriad ways from our own. This can cause problems that may be catastrophic.

In the 1960s the sleep-inducing drug thalidomide was taken by many European women, as it was approved early on by the European regulatory agencies. Thalidomide had been extensively tested, including studies on pregnant rabbits, and it was found not to cause birth defects.[2] Unfortunately rabbits are different enough from humans that the destructive effects of the drug were missed. This resulted in an epidemic of birth defects, principally a condition known as phocomelia, in which the arms and legs of the affected individual may be seriously deformed or missing. Fortunately, the FDA had not approved thalidomide, so we were saved from this tragedy. Today animal testing is much more refined, but there still are risks associated with generalizing to humans from animal data. Rats, mice and rabbits present serious shortcomings as a model for evaluating drugs.

Animal models have been greatly improved since the 1960s. The development of gene transfer technologies has enabled the engineering of rats and mice that have important human genes engineered into their genome, such as receptors on the cell surfaces that can bind human signaling proteins. Many different rat and mouse strains have been developed which carry genes for human genetic diseases. A major triumph

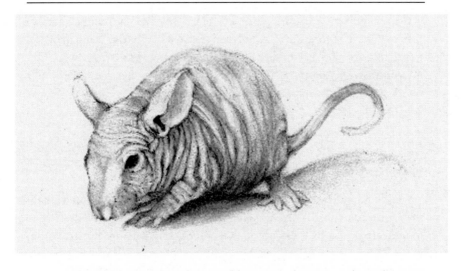

Figure 9. The nude mouse. Bizarre, resembling a tiny rhinoceros, the nude mouse has become one of the most potent research tools in cancer research. It lacks a functional immune system, and so accepts grafts of foreign tissue, including human tumor cells. For this reason it is one of the leading pre-clinical models for the evaluation of anti-cancer therapies. Drawing by Elise Morrow.

in the development of animal models was the construction of the "nude mouse," the designation referring to the animal's lack of hair, as shown in Figure 9. Nude mice, which look like tiny rhinoceroses, lack a functional immune system, so they will accept grafts of tissue from many different species. They are frequently employed to test the growth of human tumor cells. "Transgenic" mice that are engineered to carry genes from other species are so widely employed today that every large research institute has their own facility for producing them. These advances have made animal models in the 21st century a much more valuable and flexible tool for basic research.

Primates are in use today, mainly macaques and other monkeys.[3] There is growing pressure to restrict their use. They are extremely expensive to maintain, and there are severe ethical considerations in working with highly intelligent animals that clearly experience pain in the same way humans do. Any experimental plan involving the use of DNA technology supported by a federal grant must be approved by an institutional biosafety committee, composed of staff and community representatives. Federal restrictions regarding the care of primates, especially chimps, include requirements for a humane and quality environment (whatever this is). These regulations have driven the costs of maintaining primates to astronomical levels, and they are only employed as a last resort. The mountains of regulations along with the ethical issues are leading to a phase out of all primate research.[4]

Human Trials: Difficulties Threading the Needle

The most direct and accurate way to study the response of humans to hazardous substances and therapies would be through the use of humans exposed to these agents, or clinical trials using human volunteers. Since it is unethical to expose human subjects to known toxic substances, the usual approach is to follow populations that encountered these chemicals due to happenstance, or because they intentionally exposed themselves to these substances, as is the case for cigarette smokers.

This approach is fraught with problems, so it is not surprising that it is very difficult to obtain reliable, repeatable data. For example, say we wish to test the hypothesis that a particular insecticide that we apply to our skin is an "epimutagen." We will have to assemble two populations that are identical in every way, except one uses the insecticide on a regular basis, and one does not. But isn't this impossible? If an individual uses an insecticide, they have certain views and priorities about their life and their health, and this would probably mean that there are other patterns of behavior that they follow.

Another problem is that we will have to rely on their honesty and memory when we ask them how much and how long were they exposed to the agent. But ordinarily people forget, or cover up actions that they believe others do not find acceptable. Try questioning people about their alcohol consumption, smoking habits, sexual peccadillos or drug abuse and see how reliable your data are.

Then we will have to follow them for a long time, and we will have to monitor all their medical parameters. As you can see right away, this is quite similar to the atomic bomb casualty studies, and we know that even after years of study and millions of dollars in cost, we still are unable to make a definitive statement concerning the ability of radiation to cause mutations in the human genome.

A further difficulty with this sort of study is that it must be analyzed through the use of statistics, and such analyses can be complex and full of pitfalls.[5] This is a perfect example of "never try this at home." With complex studies it is absolutely essential to have the resources of a good professional statistician available, which doesn't always happen. The extent of the problem can be appreciated by statements from the Merck pharmaceutical company, whose scientists stated that they were able to confirm less than half of the studies of drug compounds published by academic research teams. There are many reasons for such appalling results, but certainly the use of flawed or improper statistical analysis is a large part of the problem.

Finally, clinical studies are required when new drugs are tested for their safety and ability to cure or alleviate a certain disease state. Today there are many studies being pursued with drugs that inhibit epigenetic processes; almost all these trials involve anti-cancer drugs. Clinical trials of this sort are carried out at three levels, phases I, II and III. These reflect the sample size, and the confidence of the investigators. Phase I trials may involve as few as a dozen patients, whereas a large scale Phase III trial can take in hundreds of patients. Once again, the result must be analyzed statistically, and there must be a group who receive the drug, and an identical group that are exposed to a placebo.

And again, there are the same sorts of caveats that apply. The statistics must be impeccable. The patients must be carefully monitored by all sorts of testing. The two groups must be perfectly randomly selected, and their identity unknown to the researchers until after the study is completed. Long followup times may be required before cryptic damage comes to the surface.

A Doorway to the Truth

These are the tools that scientists have available. You may think that they are so beset with problems that it would be surprising if they ever worked at all. But you couldn't be more wrong. This is because the scientific community has been grappling with these challenges for years, sometimes successfully, sometimes not. Over and over again studies are repeated, debated, analyzed for errors and accepted or finally rejected. To take one example, death rates from breast cancer declined by 2.2 percent per year between 1990 and 2007. Overall, between 1971 and 2007 ten year survival rates for cancer victims increased from 23.7 to 45.2 percent. These are amazing data. It is due to the development of new treatments, all achieved through the use of the methods that we have outlined above. Today longevity and quality of life are immensely improved for sufferers from this disease. So while these methods are slow, cumbersome, expensive and prone to failure, they do work. By pursuing them doggedly, obsessively, again and again, they have produced amazing benefits over a long time frame.

Professor Peter Johnson, of the Southampton Cancer Research UK Centre, said: "There are many reasons for our continuing success in the fight against cancer, including faster diagnosis, better surgery, more effective radiotherapy and many new drugs, all developed using the knowledge that our laboratory research has given us."[6]

What happens when we apply these tools to the science of epigenetics? This is the critical question, as without reliable scientific data, our whole story collapses. Let's put it to the test.

Epigenetics and Cancer: Do We Really Want to Know What's Out There?

Centuries of Struggle

"You know, John, I was in a history of medicine museum in Cardiff, and I noticed that many of the instruments that the Roman physicians used for cancer surgery were identical with those that we have today in our surgery suites."

South Texas is famous for its blistering hot summers which drive its residents into the nearest air conditioned watering hole during the heat of the day. Some years back I was doing a sabbatical, working with a breast cancer research group at the University of Texas Medical Center in San Antonio. A lot of the pleasure of this experience came from the collegiality of an international group of people working in cancer research and treatment, mostly directed toward an understanding of the way that hormones affect breast cancer. We had many long discussions of our interests in cancer and scientific discoveries over lunches at glacially air conditioned hamburger joints near the Medical Center. This comment was made by a colleague of mine, a breast cancer surgeon, Dr. Robert Mansel. "From their writings, we know that they were successful in removing tumors, if they hadn't spread to other parts of the body." Mansel, who is from Wales, spent a year in San Antonio and returned to a distinguished career in his native land.

Of course without sterile procedures or anesthetics, surgery was a dicey possibility at best, and the fact that anyone ever survived is quite a testament to the fortitude of the patients and the skill of their physicians. Because the average lifespan was so short, cancer certainly wasn't as common as it is in modern society. But since the patients were usually fairly young, they were more likely to withstand the rigors of the experience, even if their subsequent recovery was much in doubt. We know that some did survive, because the Roman physicians kept careful records.[1]

But certainly cancer was widespread. Today it is recognized that 80 to 90 percent of cancers are caused by chemicals, dietary factors and other environmental insults. In the Greco-Roman world there were innumerable industrial processes that used mercury, lead, arsenic and many other substances that we know today are extremely carcinogenic.

For centuries virtually no progress was made in our understanding of disease; throughout the Middle Ages Europe was mired in fear and superstition, and much of the medical advances made by the Greeks, Romans and Egyptians were lost. Illness and disease were looked upon by the Catholic Church as just punishments for a life ill spent; plagues and epidemics were blamed on the Jews, always a convenient scapegoat.

I mention my conversations on the history of medicine because they drove home to me how long cancer has been with us, and how tortuous the road to an understanding of this malady has been. Even today surgery is one of the first options for its treatment. And until the 20th century, it was the only option. Physicians had many medicinal compounds at their disposal, but there was no systematic way of evaluating them, and few had any effect whatsoever.

This picture gradually changed as diet and public health measures improved and the average lifespan increased throughout the industrialized world. The dark side of this picture was the emergence of diseases associated with aging and bad lifestyle choices. Today about 23 percent of all deaths in the U.S. are from cancer. And, unless there are unforeseen changes, the number of cancers will continue to increase as the population grows and as people continue to live longer. The total cost of cancer treatment was $124 billion in 2010 and it is anticipated to rise dramatically in the coming years.[2]

As we mentioned in the last chapter, the three methods of treatment today are surgery, radiation and anti-cancer drugs, and these will continue to be the available options for the foreseeable future.

What Is Cancer?

Most people recognize that cancer is some sort of uncontrolled growth process, and they may be aware of the fact that it really is a whole family of diseases, affecting different parts of the body in different ways. They are probably also conscious of the fact that there are many different treatments and many different outcomes. We're not going to go into the clinical details of various cancers here; there are many sources that do this, and so many people have had encounters with cancer that they may already have a fair amount of knowledge regarding its clinical attributes. Here we're going to talk about the genetic/epigenetic connection and why this is so critical for our understanding of this illness.

Today cancer researchers know a great deal about their subject. Although the details of the picture change from day to day as new findings are collected and interpreted, our overall understanding is solid, and firmly in place. It is as follows.

Cancer is a disorder of cellular control mechanisms. It is caused by a failure of the organism to regulate normal growth and division. It is due to changes in one or more genes that produce molecules that control these processes. There are many such controlling genes and more are constantly being discovered. In their normal state they are known as proto-oncogenes, and when they move to the dark side through alterations, known as mutations, they become oncogenes. In some instances they are carried into the body by viruses, in which case they are referred to as viral oncogenes.[3] There are also genes that control the expression of oncogenes. Under ordinary conditions they form a vast regulatory network, operating smoothly, talking back and forth to one another and keeping their owners in a state of stability, if not of bliss.

In the 1970s it was suspected that perhaps all cancers were caused by viruses, either directly, by bringing in an oncogene, or indirectly by causing inflammation or other disruptive processes that favored the growth of cancer cells. This was the belief that drove the Nixon administration's War on Cancer in the early 1970s, a costly and unfortunate failure. Since many viral diseases, especially polio, had been eliminated through vaccination, it was believed that in the same way cancer could be cured through a cancer vaccine. Sadly, this proved not to be true, and after years of effort and billions of dollars the program was abandoned.

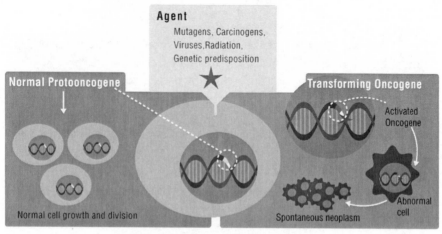

Agent
Mutagens, Carcinogens,
Viruses,Radiation,
Genetic predisposition

Normal Protooncogene

Transforming Oncogene

Activated
Oncogene

Abnormal
cell

Normal cell growth and division

Spontaneous neoplasm

The Dual Nature of Oncogene

Figure 10. The oncogene. Oncogenes are genes which in their normal state (the proto-oncogene) regulate growth and cellular behavior. Agents in the environment (chemicals, radiation, stress, hormones) can cause changes in the DNA or can affect epigenetic control mechanisms. The result is that the proto-oncogene does not follow its normal pattern, and the cell's growth becomes unregulated, resulting in abnormal proliferation. In many cases, the tumor does not remain confined to its original site within the body, but breaks apart, forming secondary tumors in other locations (metastasis). Drawing by Garima Naredi.

Today it is generally accepted that around 5 percent of all cancers in industrialized countries are caused by viruses, although in some countries the figure may be as high as 20 percent.[4] There are vaccines available for the human papilloma virus (HPV), the major cause of cervical cancer. But such vaccines attack a specific virus, and in the majority of cancers, no specific virus can be detected, even after years of searching.

Numerous research programs are studying therapies that bolster the immune system so it wards off cancers, and these have met with some success. There is, at long last, a vaccine approved by the FDA for the treatment of prostate cancer, known as Provenge. It is nothing like a conventional vaccine such as that for polio or the HPV vaccine. In the case of Provenge, immune cells are removed from the patient, exposed to prostate antigens, and re-introduced. However, its use has been marred by bitter controversy, including death threats against physicians that argued against its approval.[5] Recent studies show that it provides some months of increased survival for prostate cancer patients whose cancers have spread.[6]

Currently a large clinical trial is underway testing a cancer vaccine, known as L-BLP25,[7] in which patients are immunized with a protein called MUC-1, a protein which is overproduced in colon cancer cells. It will be months or years before a decision can be made regarding performance. But even if these experiments are successful, it is highly unlikely that a universal vaccine is possible, or even a family of vaccines that could immunize us against all cancers, eliminating cancer in the same fashion that made polio a thing of the past.

It takes mutations in many of the oncogenes to bring about the transformation to malignancy. This is why cancer is a slow, step by step process. We can see this in lung cancer, which is the most frequent type of cancer and perhaps the most intensively studied. It is almost entirely due to cigarette smoking. Despite the filth and dreadful pollution of 19th century industrialized America, lung cancer was virtually unknown. In the early 20th century cigarettes were adopted by society as a less smelly alternative to cigars, beginning around 1900. Cigar smoke is so alkaline that it cannot be drawn into the lungs, whereas cigarette smoke may be inhaled. The incidence of smoking, only among men, increased rapidly until it peaked at about 50 percent of the adult population in the early 1960s.

About 30 years or so of enthusiastic cigarette consumption are needed to bring on a case of lung cancer, so it did not begin to appear in men until the 1930s. Women started smoking in large numbers about 30 years later, and so their lung cancer rates did not start to go up until the 1960s. When smoke is inhaled, the cells of the lungs are bathed in a concentrated solution of carcinogens every day for hours on end. Starting slowly, one proto-oncogene after another falls, like a row of dominos, and over the years the lung tissue gradually becomes more and more abnormal and distorted. The tissue loses its coherence, and instead of consisting of neat, orderly rows of cells, it appears more and more unruly and disorganized. The process feeds back upon itself, until the entire hereditary makeup of the cell is destabilized, driving more genes to mutate. You can see this in microscopic samples of tissues taken from smokers who died of unrelated causes, and now with DNA sequencing technology you can follow the genetic alterations in the DNA of the oncogenes in the cancerous cells that we know are responsible for lung cancer. With advances in the technology, it is now possible to follow precancerous lesion by sampling tissues obtained with bronchoscopy and analyzing the material through a variety of special stains.[8]

Myths, Fantasies, Realities

This might be a good time to consider some of the myths and realities concerning cancer, since they are widespread. We need to rid ourselves of these misconceptions if we are to appreciate the role that epigenetics plays in cancer.

1. The first and most egregious is that **there is a cure for cancer that is being hidden by the cancer establishment**. This is one that drives my daughter-in-law, an oncologist, up the wall. She even hears this from some of her employees, that there is a mysterious cure for cancer, hidden by some vast conspiracy. Like all conspiracy theories, this one defies common sense. Cancer is not *a* disease, it is a family of diseases. I'm not going to list the alphabet soup of all the proto-oncogenes that are known, but one census that I inspected details about 300, and there are probably many more. Furthermore, scientists have estimated that for any individual cancer there may be as many as 80 different oncogenes that are taking part in the process. Since they perform a whole range of tasks when operating in their normal mode, there is no possibility of *a* cure. There could only be myriad cures.

The granddaddy of all cancer conspiracy claims regards a character by the unlikely name of Royal Raymond Rife, who, in the 1930s designed a mysterious device that he claimed produced "energetically exciting destructive resonances in the constituent chemicals of cancer cells." In the decades following Rife's announcement there have been innumerable claims that his cure for cancer was suppressed by a greedy medical establishment that was desperately trying to protect its gold mine of dying cancer patients.[9] Garbage science dies hard: as recently as 2009 a purveyor of "Rife Machines" was sent to prison.

But say there were a single cure, hidden by the cancer establishment, in opposition to all reason? Is there any way this information could be suppressed, year after year after year? Since cancer is so ubiquitous, wouldn't the people in control of this magical treatment want to use it on themselves? And why wouldn't they want to come out of the closet, sell the cure and make a fortune and win a Nobel Prize? And finally, why do people who put their trust in physicians and scientists believe the medical establishment could be so cruel and pernicious as to sacrifice the lives of millions of people, including their own, simply so they could keep secret the biggest discovery in the history of science?

2. **You can cure yourself of cancer by willing it.** If you frame this as a question on the Internet you'll get about 3.5 million responses, so it's obvious that a lot people believe that you can overcome cancer just by a positive attitude. Furthermore there are all sorts of stories written by people who claim that diet, exercise, prayer and a host of other lifestyle modifications saved their lives. These stories are invariably testimonies by people stating that the doctors had given up on them, they had months to live, until they happened upon a wondrous cure.[10] The doctors were astonished, they were confounded, they had stated unequivocally that the author of the website had days or weeks or months to live. Often these people offer books, programs and other paraphernalia to disarm the unwary.

Sadly these websites rarely have anything, other than anecdotal evidence, to support their claims. In cases in which such "miracle cures" have actually been tested, they invariably fall flat. There are innumerable examples of celebrities who desperately wanted to live, tried every bizarre cure regime under the sun, and invariably died. The National Institute for Complementary and Alternative Medicine is a federal agency that was formed in an effort to add some scientific analysis to this contentious area. They have investigated many of these treatments, and they have never been able to find an authentic alternative cure. As might be imagined, there are harsh critics of the Institute on both sides of the question. Detractors claim that the institute has wasted $800 million since its founding in 1991.

There are rare people diagnosed with cancers by reputable medical experts who recover without chemotherapy or other conventional treatments. What are we do think about this? Two types of cancer, neuroblastoma and melanoma, have been observed to disappear in this fashion as we discussed previously. We'll have more to say about that later on, but this type of behavior is precisely the way we expect epigenetically controlled traits to act; unstable, rapidly changing and hard to predict.

But the great albatross around the neck of the institute is the fact that it was founded to test all these claims, and given the cost and complexity of clinical trials, one could hardly expect it to succeed. When people participate in a clinical trial of an anti cancer drug, they must be thoroughly monitored, a processes costing thousands of dollars per patient. All of their vital signs and responses are tested over and over again, and hundreds of physicians and other medical personnel will be required to take part. Just to give you a feeling of the size of the problem, Genentech, a major biotech company has spent several billion dollars (yes, that's billion with a B!) testing Avastin, a big blockbuster drug used to treat several forms of cancer. So it's not surprising that the Institute has satisfied virtually no one in its efforts to complete its mission.

This is not the place to thoroughly evaluate such a politically charged question. But we can certainly conclude that all the solid scientific evidence available at this time has not produced a shred of evidence supporting the value of alternative treatments for cancer. If such treatments are of any value, the burden of proof rests on those who would make such a claim.

3. **There are wonder treatments for cancer that the U.S. regulatory agencies won't allow, that you can obtain in foreign countries.** Once again, if you go on the Internet you will find many clinics in China, Mexico and other foreign countries that offer amazing treatments for cancer that you cannot obtain in the U.S. And there is a good reason that you cannot obtain them here. It is because there is no solid evidence that they work, and no proof that they are safe. Keep in mind that laws are very different in China, that China is pushing biotechnology very aggressively, that the society is completely opaque, and that you have absolutely no legal recourse if things go wrong. Most of these companies are closely associated with the Chinese government, which has every reason to be lax on enforcement of high standards of drug efficacy and safety. Moreover, there are no laws to protect whistleblowers (in fact it is the other way around; whistleblowers are routinely punished) and there is no freedom of expression in China. Moreover, the cost of these treatments is very high, as are the costs of travel and the associated living expenses.

All the other locations that you find on the Internet are in foreign countries that have lax or non-existent regulation of medical care. This doesn't mean that you cannot obtain first class health care through medical tourism to Singapore, Mexico, India or Thailand. There are clinics in these countries that offer first world medicine, administered by staff trained and board certified in the U.S., offering a wide range of medical care for much less than what an uninsured patient would be hit with in the U.S. But if you encounter claims of an astounding cure that sounds too good to be true, well, it no doubt is too good to be true.

I have looked for peer reviewed publications in high profile scientific journals on one of these treatments offered in China, called Genticine, and I find none. Does this mean that alternative medicine is a complete failure, that travel to foreign countries for therapies is a waste, that there are no routes to safe and effective treatment except through conventional U.S. medicine? Not necessarily. I could be wrong. It simply means that the burden of proof is on the groups marketing these treatments, and if they want to convince skeptics, they need powerful and well documented evidence. When our lives are in the balance, I don't think this is asking too much.

4. **A cure for cancer is right around the corner.** This is a common misconception, often promoted by scientists, university media departments, drug companies and other players with a big stake in the game. "We will cure cancer in your lifetime" is a common mantra. It's not that these folks are dishonest or trying to deceive you, they're simply forced into a business model that requires that they come out with encouraging statements all the time. If they didn't, the public would lose patience and would quit supporting them. They would quit voting for politicians that support large federal research budgets and they would quit buying drug company stocks.[11]

It's important to remember that if an encouraging basic research discovery is made in a scientist's laboratory, it will be, on the average, 15 years before a new drug emanating from this discovery is available to the public. That's because it will have to proceed through many levels of testing before it can even be entered into clinical trials, and clinical trials can take years. Just to give you a personal example, an acquaintance of mine is CEO of a biopharma company that has been testing their anti-cancer drugs for 20 years, without satisfying the FDA, the regulatory agency that approves new therapies.

It should be noted that although surgery, chemotherapy and radiation are the traditional options for cancer treatment, their performance over the years has been less than stellar. These treatments are often devastating and painful, and in the case of many cancers add little life extension to the patient. A widely quoted study carried out in the U.S. and Australia found that the five year survival for all patients was about 63 percent but that chemotherapy contributed only 2 percent to this result. This abysmal record is largely due to the fact that most cancers are solid tumors which respond poorly to chemotherapy. The record is much better for circulating cancers, which are a small fraction of total cases.

Another big problem with cancer treatment is that vast resources are focused on terminal patients in the last months of life. At this point the cancers have metastasized (or spread) to other regions of the body, and the likelihood of a cure is very small. Antibodies are the drug du jour for cancer treatment these days. For instance, Herceptin, an anticancer antibody, extends the lives of stomach cancer patients on the average by three months,[12] at an annual cost of $54,000.

But when we look at the global picture, including a whole range of patients and tumor types, we certainly can see reason for optimism. For patients sampled between 1975 and 1977, the overall five year survival rate for all cancers was 49 percent. In the aggregate 2001–2007 group, that figure had risen to 67 percent.[13] And survival does not take into account the fact that quality of life for cancer patients has vastly improved, which is much harder to quantify. Surgery is much less invasive and traumatic, chemotherapy treatments are less devastating, radiation is delivered by sophisticated, computer-driven devices that produce a narrow, targeted beam of radiation that causes much less damage to surrounding tissues.

This is what we have to look forward to: small, incremental gains from year, brought about by discoveries in the basic sciences and their application to treatments established through endless, expensive and laborious testing.

I believe there is no alternative to this gloomy prediction.

The Discovery of the Oncogene[14]

We come back to cancer and epigenetics again, because oncology is currently on the forefront of epigenetic research. There are even four "epigenetic" drugs approved by the FDA, and there are many more in various stages of development. All of these drugs are anti-cancer drugs, so this is the area of epigenetics that shows the most promise at this time. But it also shows great risks. As we will see, other dark alleys that we will explore within the epigenetic landscape may be even more threatening.

As we mentioned previously, cancer was for many years believed to result from mutations in the DNA of normal cells that altered oncogenes controlling growth and cell division patterns. Oncogene research was put on a solid footing in the 1970s. The first known oncogene was christened "SRC," named after the Rous sarcoma virus from which it was isolated. The virus, which occurs in chickens, causes a cancer found in soft tissue, referred to as a sarcoma. In one of the early triumphs of recombinant gene manipulation, the section of the viral genetic material that could produce a tumor was isolated and sequenced. It turned out that the SRC viral gene is very similar to a gene occurring in humans that codes for a growth promoting enzyme, tyrosine kinase.

SRC opened the door to the discovery of a whole rogue's gallery of oncogenes, since it is but one of a family of similar enzymes. As more tools for manipulation of DNA were discovered and perfected, it became easier and faster to move genes around, to sequence them and study their myriad properties. Some of the new oncogenes that were uncovered are similar to SRC, whereas others are completely unrelated. As more and more oncogenes were carefully studied, a variety of changes were found that led to a cancerous transformation. These oncogenes could become unhinged from their regulators, producing more and more of their growth promoting products. Or in some cases an oncogene could be duplicated over and over again, so many copies of a normal gene were pumping out more and more of a growth promoter. Yet other circumstances involved a gene that suppressed growth that became nonfunctional. Without its dampening effect growth becomes disturbed, and the cell proliferates wildly.[15]

The Cancer Connection: The Devil in the Details

The field has changed dramatically in recent years, as research on epigenetics and cancer has morphed into a booming research endeavor.

In the early days of the human genome project only limited success was encountered in the hunt for new cancer related genes. There has been much attention paid to the breast cancer related mutations, BRCA1 and BRCA2. Individuals with these mutated genes have a greatly elevated risk of breast and ovarian cancer. But it turns out that these DNA-based mutations are only responsible for a small fraction of cancers, maybe 2 percent. So this leaves a great gap in our understanding of the basis of all these other cancers.

You can imagine the excitement when researchers found epigenes that were involved in tumorigenesis. Animal studies and experiments with tissue culture cells showed that some drugs that cause methylation will suppress genes that are identified as tumor suppressing genes. Thus, two negatives make a positive, and the cells behave as tumor cells. This means that they can form tumors when injected into appropriate lab animals and that they fulfill other criteria of cancer cells.

How do these observations fit into a theory or an overall picture of the origins of cancer?

The current view that is emerging is that both mutations in the DNA code and epigenetic changes to regions of the DNA that affect the reading of the genetic messages produce cancers. They may both occur in certain tumors, and a number of these changes over time push the cell into a more and more abnormal state. In fact, in the case of neuroendocrine tumors, scientists have found that as much as 60 percent of the patients with neuroendocrine tumors have epigenetic changes and 40 percent of kidney cancer patients show these alterations. In note number 1, Chapter 14, I provide some details on megaprojects that the NIH has underway to understand the cancer epigenome.

Epigenetic changes can drive cancers in another way. Recently a bizarre cancer has been destroying a rare marsupial, the Tasmanian devil.[16] This animal is a canine-like creature and lives entirely on the Australian island of Tasmania. The cancer, which first appeared in the 1980s, is distinguished by tumors around the mouths of the animals, and cells from these tumors are transmitted by biting when the animals encounter one another. The tumors spread around the mouth and larynx, restricting the breathing and feeding of the devils, causing their demise. Because the animals are very similar to each other from a genetic standpoint, the cells passed during this biting process are not recognized as foreign by the animal's immune system and are essentially a graft of cancer cells. Recent studies indicate that the tumor cells are epigenetically unhinged and are capable of evolving rapidly and adapting to altered conditions. By transmission from animal to animal the cells have become immortalized, living long after their host have died. Because of the epigenetic plasticity of these tumors they have become more aggressive in the course of their transmission from animal to animal. Currently there are breeding programs in place in an attempt to develop animals whose immune system can recognize the transmitted tumor cells as foreign and prevent them from establishing themselves in the infected animal.

The miserable situation in which the Tasmanian devil finds itself is fortunately rare, though not unique. We never think of cancer as an infectious disease, yet there are cases in humans in which cancer can be transmitted from one individual to another. The best known and best understood is HPV or human papilloma infection, a sexually transmitted condition, in which a virus causes cervical carcinoma and other cancers of the reproductive system. But this cancer is transmitted by the virus, not by the infected cells. Because humans are so genetically diverse, no two are exactly identical (even identical twins!) and foreign cells will be recognized and rejected out of hand. Thus the vast majority of human cancers cannot be spread from person to person.

There are two important questions that must be answered if we are to accept the concept of environmental epimutagens as a major force in cancer causation. First, are epigenetic changes implicated in a major portion of human cancers and secondly, are these epigenetic alterations caused by substances (referred to as "epimutagens") in our environment? I believe that both these questions can be answered in the affirmative.

First, extremely sophisticated molecular techniques are now revealing profound alterations in the "epigenome" of cancer cells that accompany the changes in the DNA of the genome that have been recognized for so long. This has been observed over and over again in cancer cells; in some cases virtually all of the cancer cells examined shows changes in their epigenome. Dr. Stephen Baylin, a leading epigenetics investigator at Johns Hopkins University, talks of "myriad abnormalities" in cells of many different cancers that can be passed on to descendent cells. In several types of cancer that have been thoroughly studied, two genes that

71

suppress tumor formation are turned off by epigenetic changes, meaning that the control of normal cell growth has been interrupted, and tumor cell growth can proceed without restraint. In both Wilm's tumor (a kidney cancer) and in colon cancer, the earliest changes seen in the cells are epigenetic in nature. In the case of some cancers, mutations in the DNA occur in genes that control epigenetic processes. So an interplay exists, with genome mutations in the DNA disrupting normal growth and control, and affecting genes that control epigenomic processes. These activities work back and forth as the tissues slides down the road to greater and greater abnormality.

There are many, many examples of the epigenetic connection from studies in the laboratory using animals or tissues culture cells in addition to innumerable observations on human subjects. A conclusive proof of this dance of death carried on between the genome and the epigenome is the fact that chemical agents that reverse epigenetic changes are now employed in cancer treatment. The work is in its early stages, but it is clear that the strategy can offer important benefits for cancer patients.[17]

How a Toxic Environment Causes Epigenetic Damage

Scientists are building a clear and detailed picture of how damage to the epigenome occurs. I am going to present a number of lines of evidence that establish in an undeniable fashion that chemicals producing epigenetic damage are a widespread source of a host of debilitating conditions. When scientists measure the effects of any agent on a biological system, a rule that must be persistently observed is that the more of the agent fed into the system, the greater the effect. Of course at a certain point you would expect to reach a saturation level, beyond which you would not see an increasing effect, and in fact you might see a decrease, as the agent blocked itself, in the manner of a queue, in which the people in the line mob each other and the whole forward movement grinds to a halt. So if you didn't see more of the effect as you increased the dose, then the cause-and-effect relationship would be highly suspect.

Another concern that scientists face when evaluating suspect agents is whether the amount of a substance found to be highly active at high doses in a laboratory setting has any relevant effect at the much lower doses at which it might be present in the environment. We know that biological systems have the capacity to repair themselves; could it be that at very low doses there are cellular enzymes that can fix this modest amount of damage?

We saw in Chapter 3 that for years the survivors of the atomic blasts at Hiroshima and Nagasaki have been evaluated periodically. We also found that while there has been some increase in rates of leukemia in these folks, there is no evidence that mutations were increased in the children or grandchildren of the survivors. This could mean that there is a threshold for damage to the genetic material from radiation or other agents in the environment, and this could apply to both epigenetic and genetic damage. Or it could mean that the dose received by the human populations that have been monitored so far was simply too low to cause a measurable amount of damage. In either case the message is clear: if we want to draw a cause and effect relation between epimutagens and an increase in disease, your science needs to be airtight.

Recently, some very nice studies have published by an international team who looked at Benzene exposure and DNA methylation in Bulgarian petroleum workers.[18] Benzene is a powerful carcinogen, closely linked to such cancers as acute myeloid leukemia. The investigators found that the greater the exposure to benzene, the greater the amount of hypomethylation in their DNA. So these kinds of studies show that an especially toxic environment can produce the epigenetic changes in DNA that we know are associated with cancer causation. The authors caution that the correlation was a weak one, hardly surprising when we think of all the intervening factors that could distort the analysis.

Cigarettes: A Good Starting Point

The best place to begin our consideration of epimutagens is with cigarette smoking, since the doses of cancer-causing compounds that the smoker receives are so high that if you didn't see a strong effect here, you would have to throw out the whole idea. And this has proven to be a fruitful area of study. A mountain of research data has shown that many chemicals present in cigarette smoke can behave as epimutagens.

These chemicals include some really bad actors, such as N-nitrosamine, 4-(methylnitrasomino)-1-(-pyridyl)-1-butanone, and a raft of other substances. These molecules behave as mutagens, but they also act as epimutagens, and now their effects can be separated. While they have been tested on tissue culture cells and lab animals, the most definitive evidence come from smoking-induced epigenetic events observed in the clinic. Tissue samples taken from the lungs of cigarette smokers show hypermethylated promoters in both smokers with and without active cancers.[19] Recall that when these promoters sites are decorated with methyl groups, the genes that they control are shut down, and these include cancer suppressing genes. And, significantly, the degree of methylation increases with the heavy smokers. But the amount of methylation decreases in former smokers. Since genetic mutations are more or less permanent and epigenetic changes are reversible, this may explain why former smokers have lower cancer rates than current smokers. A final, powerful piece of evidence is the fact that heavy smokers who remained cancer free (we all know these people) had less methylation of the suspect genes than did heavy smokers who received the losing lottery ticket.

Recent studies of lung tissue taken from smokers have shown large increases in methylation of specific genes known to be tumor suppressor genes; in one study there was a three fold increase in methylation of a tumor suppressor gene associated with a common lung cancer, non small cell lung carcinoma. In fact, DNA methylation of specific genes is such a consistent indication of cancer risk that screening tests have been developed using DNA methylation status of genes in cells taken from the plasma of at-risk patients.

One of the most disturbing observations to rear its ugly head in recent years is the fact that when a large number of toxic chemicals are selected at random and tested for their ability to cause cancer, a large percentage, usually around half, turn up positive. And of these, around 40 percent, or 20 percent of the total do not cause mutations in the DNA. We must assume that most, probably all, are working through epigenetic mechanisms. There have been many studies of this type. Some work has been done on people with bladder cancers, which are associated with exposure to second hand smoke. The tumors of these individuals have a high level of DNA methylation in a number of cancer-related genes. There are many, many studies of this type, and whereas the numbers vary somewhat, they're all close together.

So what can we conclude? That cigarettes, powerful delivery systems for carcinogenic chemicals, cause both epigenetic and genetic changes in cells that over time result in a variety of cancers. That the levels of these chemicals are more than enough to produce a whole range of different types of cancers. That there is an interplay between the genetic and the epigenetic effects. All these lines of evidence make a strong case for the lethality of cigarettes.[20]

There's Bad News and Then There's Bad News

Many folks reading this are going to react by saying, "That's all well and good, but I don't smoke, and I'm not around smokers or cigarettes, so this doesn't affect me. Just because you can make a powerful and convincing argument for epigenetic mechanisms as the driver for their cancer-causing ability, that only shows that very high doses of epimutagens, taken over a long period (years!) can cause cancer. Probably the amounts of these chemicals that the average non-smoker is exposed to are so low that their effects are trivial, or even non-existent, if the threshold concept is really accurate."

Besides, the doubters can argue, if this were true, that low doses of epigenetic chemicals are causing increases in cancer rates: Shouldn't we see this? Shouldn't there be big spikes in cancer incidences? Aren't cancer rates actually going down?

These are all important questions, and they deserve thoughtful answers, because now we are getting into an extremely controversial area, the effect of man-made modifications to our world on human health. This debate has been going on for years, but now it takes on new significance. Back in the 1960s, when the dispute over environmental destruction started heating up, most of the dispute was over pollutants that caused immediate damage to bodily functions, such as damage to the heart, lungs and other organs. There wasn't a lot of discussion of changes to the genome or the epigenome because no such words had entered into public usage. As we discussed earlier, neither the scientific framework nor the technical tools for studying the genomics-epigenomics structure had been invented.

Nowadays this is all changed. Scientists are starting to look at some chemicals that may be epimutagens that are widespread in our environment. Let's start out with a group of compounds known as "endocrine disruptors." These chemicals mimic natural hormones and interfere with their functions. The most widespread is BPA, a chemical used in the manufacture of plastic drink and food containers and in the epoxy resins that coat food and drink cans. Virtually everyone in the world that lives in an industrial environment has detectable levels of BPA in their urine, and for a long time the sole concern of environmental scientists was the possibility that BPA and the hundreds of other related endocrine disruptors to which we are exposed could interfere with natural hormones, and disrupt normal reproductive functions. But now a growing body of evidence points to these substances as powerful epimutagens. These experiments, performed on animals and tissue culture cells, show that BPA can cause methylation (the best measure of epigenetic effects) in breast epithelial cells at very low concentrations, comparable to those observed in human fetuses.[21] But there are many other disturbing observations. These same concentrations of BPA can cause changes in the microRNA molecules known for their involvement in several types of malignant cancers.

We can add lots of other bad actors to this growing list. One of the worst is Vinclozolin, a fungicide and endocrine disruptor long used in vineyards, golf courses and on fruit and vegetable crops. Fortunately its use has been restricted, but it is still used on golf course turf and canola fields.

At the beginning of this chapter I called attention to the widespread use of metals in Greco-Roman industrial processes, taking note of their carcinogenicity. For instance, nickel compounds have long been known to cause cancer, although they do not cause mutations in the DNA. But they do cause methylation changes and can shut down genes so that they don't produce cancer suppressors. Cadmium and chromium cause methylation changes in the promoter genes that regulate cancer suppressors. Lead is widely distributed in the environment and is associated with cancer causation and methylation. Arsenic, the old friend of mystery writers, is also a powerful epimutagen, but does not cause mutations in the DNA.

You may be surprised to learn this (I certainly was!), but asbestos continues to be mined and exported from the U.S., even though it has long been known to cause mesothelioma, a particularly nasty form of lung cancer. Asbestos is banned in the European Union, though it is still permitted in the U.S. in the construction of asbestos pipes. It is believed that around 2000 tons of asbestos were released during the destruction of the World Trade Center on 9/11.[22] Patients with mesothelioma who were exposed to asbestos have a high incidence (almost 100 percent) of methylation of tumor suppressor genes.[23]

Lots of people enjoy the "new car smell"; this is due to a number volatile compounds vaporizing out of the materials (especially the upholstery) that comprise a new automobile. When the vehicle is right off the assembly line, these chemicals come pouring out, especially phthalates, or plasticizers. And guess what? These are epimutagens, so you might want to think about a used car instead. Regardless of how good it smells, after three weeks, 90 percent of the aerosol disappears.

Probably the meanest, nastiest chemicals that humans have able to come up with are a class known as "polycyclic aromatic hydrocarbons." These malefactors are responsible for just about every miserable disease you could imagine. There are thousands of them; they are produced as petroleum biproducts. They are used for many industrial processes and they constitute the building blocks of pesticides. The focus of research used to be on their ability to cause mutations in the DNA (they are pretty good at it), but their real forte is as epimutagens. One study turned up over 2000 genes that were epigenetically modified, following exposure to some of these compounds.

Same old same old. As we survey the scientific literature, the pattern keeps repeating itself. Nasty molecules, banging around the environment. Studies on animals and tissue culture cells, evidence of cancers and epigenetic change. Little evidence of changes in the DNA sequences of the genome. Studies on humans, linking exposure to these substances to increases in cancer rates.

But what about cancer incidence? Shouldn't the rates of cancers be increasing if exposure to epimutagens is more and more widespread? This is a complicated question, since you need to study epimutagens in isolation from other factors, and this is extremely difficult, if not impossible. For example, around 65 percent of bladder cancer in men is attributable to cigarette smoking, which has declined over the years. So it is not surprising that overall rates of bladder cancer are lower now. And remember that I told you there is an interaction between genetic and epigenetic mechanisms. These facts make it difficult to do a meaningful study that can demonstrate an unequivocal effect in a large population.

What Goes Around...

A drive across West Texas will fulfill all your cliché-ridden notions about the Lone Star State. A sky that seems to dwarf everything beneath it, a desolate, parched prairie stretching off to the ends of the earth, scorching hot summer days and freezing winter nights. I used to take this trip on a monthly basis to confer with a colleague, Dr. Philip Periman, a hematologist in Amarillo, Texas, whose research interest was multiple myeloma.

Myeloma is a cancer of the blood, actually the antibody producing cells found in the circulation. He saw a lot of patients with this disease; at that time it was a death sentence, although it could be held at bay for some time with conventional chemotherapy. Periman was struck by its high incidence in ranchers and farmers in the Texas Panhandle. Exposure to pesticides and other farm chemicals was long suggested as a risk factor. Recent research provides a connection: these chemicals are epimutagens, and myeloma appears to be an "epigenetic cancer" that can be successfully treated with drugs that block methylation of cancer-causing genes.

Pomalidomide and lenalidomide are recently FDA-approved derivatives of thalidomide.[24] You may recall thalidomide caused devastating birth defects during the early 1960s when used as a sedative by pregnant women in Europe. But now it has been resurrected as a cancer treatment, and its derivatives, pomalidomide and lenalidomide lack the unpleasant side effects. When given to patients with multiple myeloma, they block the methylation of a critical growth-controlling gene, $p21^{WAF}$. The end result is a reversal of the cancer-causing effects of the pesticides, and a self-destructive cascade resulting in the death of the tumor cells. These drugs have been so successful that they have kept myeloma patients alive for years, revolutionizing their chances of survival.

So the path of cause and effect looks clear. Pesticides and other epimutagenic compounds methylate suicide genes, shutting them off, so the tumor cells lose control of division. This results in cancers such as myeloma which can be destroyed by reactivating the suicide pathways through drugs that cause demethylation.[25]

In the years to come we will see this as a recurrent theme in the origins and treatment of many different cancers.

Difficult Choices

The observations of cancer and its successful treatment in myeloma patients are certainly strong evidence for an important role for epigenetic mechanisms. But as a rule, studies linking cause and effect of environmental cancer-causing compounds are difficult to do. It is hard to find any group of people anywhere in the world that don't have traces of BPA in their blood. It could be that epigenetic damage happens early in fetal development; this makes sense, since fetuses are extremely sensitive to many environmental effects. Maybe when we reach adulthood we become relatively resistant to epigenetic changes. So perhaps the low levels of these substances that show up in blood aren't anything to worry about. And of course BPA isn't the only offending substance in plastics. There are many, many different compounds in plastics that soften, stiffen, protect or provide different beneficial properties. And there is a deluge of chemicals washing our environment that are of tremendous economic benefit: drugs, solvents, coloring agents, herbicides, pesticides, cosmetics, and on and on. Maybe we really don't have the body of evidence to make significant decisions, and we should wait till scientists amass an overwhelming case.

Maybe that day is here.

The message that I have received from scientists working in the field and from published accounts is that we do indeed have a powerful case for a cancer connection with epigenetics. There is a growing recognition that epigenetic damage may be introduced in very early stages of life, in embryonic development, increasing the risk of cancers much later in the life of the individual. According to Dr. Shuk-mei Ho of the University of Cincinnati, "There is an emerging consensus that early embryonic development is a time of increased susceptibility to the effects of environmental agents, and that reprogramming of the epigenome by environmental exposures early in life can determine the risk of many adult diseases, including cancer, decades before disease onset."[26]

But there are no easy choices, and the fact the scientific issues are complex does not mean that they should be ignored. Today, scientists who study environmentally-based cancers are in agreement that epigenetic damage is a significant factor in cancer causation, and the as we have discussed in this chapter, this conclusion is pretty inescapable. How much and what can we do to avoid it? Let's consider some of the other health damage from epigenetic mechanisms, and then we will look at what we do to combat it.

6

Epigenetics and Diabetes: More Grim News

"The global epidemic of type 2 diabetes mellitus is one of the most challenging problems of the 21st century."[1]—Diabetes researchers Dharambir K. Sanghera and Piers R. Blackett

Astronomical Increases in the Frequency of a Devastating Illness

Sanghera and Blackett's statement sums up this chapter. But there is so much more to say. Theirs is one of many similar admonitions, coming from scientists overwhelmed by the magnitude of the problem. The authors go on to state that diabetes is a leading cause of coronary heart disease, stroke, peripheral vascular disease, blindness, renal failure and amputation. Global health expenditures for its treatment are predicted to rise to $490 billion by 2030. These terrible statistics go on and on. There are thought to be 346 million type II diabetics worldwide, roughly 5 percent of the world population. One more frightening number: In 2006 Medicare spent $8.6 billion on kidney dialysis and associated treatment. And this number will only continue to rise in the coming years.

Obesity, a well known risk factor for diabetes, has tripled in children and adolescents since 1980. Although this is a major contributor to increasing incidence of diabetes, other risk factors including environmental chemicals, stress and micronutrients are now under consideration as contributors to its increase in the population.[2]

What Is Diabetes?

In the spirit of our "Need to Know" approach, I'm going to give you a general outline of what this disease is. As with the other complex conditions we grappled with in the book, there are many detailed and easily available sources of information describing the clinical picture of this disorder.

Diabetes is a group of diseases in which patients have high levels of blood sugar caused by lack of insulin (type I) or lack of response to insulin (type II). Type I is due to a loss or malfunction of the beta cells of the pancreas, and is treatable with insulin injections. Type II is due to insulin resistance in which cell receptors do not respond to insulin, and is treatable through a range of drug options.

Insulin is a protein molecule, one of the traffic cops, that directs the body's metabolism to bring glucose from the blood and store it as a complex sugar, glycogen, in the liver and muscles. This is all part of the body's system of feedback and regulatory controls that maintain a balanced state. When things are working the way they should, the body gets glucose by pulling glycogen from the liver and making it into glucose which is itself converted into energy. In the absence or malfunction of insulin, cells will convert fat into energy with a litany of adverse consequences.

Complications from long-term, untreated diabetes are extremely serious. These include cardiovascular disease, chronic renal failure, retinal damage, effects on fertility, and loss of limbs as a result of vessel failure. In fact, without careful control, virtually every system of the body is gravely affected.

There is no cure for diabetes. With a lifetime commitment to vigilant monitoring and management, diabetics may hope to live out a normal lifespan. This includes keeping the glucose levels as close to normal as possible using drugs, diet, exercise, refraining from smoking and other lifestyle adjustments.[3] Medication includes insulin and a wide range of drugs for the type II form. This means that diabetics must be thoroughly educated and willing to make severe adjustments to their habits and behavior in order to avoid the looming health problems associated with this condition. Unfortunately, as is the case with any extreme personal adjustment, it is frequently difficult to get diabetics to make the modifications necessary to optimize their health status.

As is true of so many of the diseases that we wrestle with in this book, the origins of diabetes are complex, starting with the two forms— type I and II—which appear to actually represent two different diseases. Both are brought on by a combination of genetic and environmental factors, but type II diabetes, which represents 85 percent of cases, has a stronger genetic basis.

We know this because twin studies have shown that when an identical twin has type II diabetes, the co-twin has a one in two chance of also having diabetes, On the other hand, for type I diabetes, if an identical twin is affected, the co-twin has only a 1 in 3 chance of also having diabetes. Twin studies have been used for more than a century to try and separate the relative contributions of heredity and environment to the sum of an individual's overall collection of characteristics, what we refer to as the person's *phenotype*. The twin study method is based on the assumption (which is not 100 percent correct) that identical twins have exactly the same genetic constitution, and therefore a totally genetically controlled trait (such as eye color) should be 100 percent concordant (or the same). That is, if one twin has it, the other twin will always have it. If, on the other hand, the two twins are not 100 percent concordant, then the environment must contribute to the discrepancy. In this case, differences in life style factors such as nutrition, exercise, smoking habits and occupation might influence the level of non-concordance through epigenetic signals (see below).

Obesity is long known to play a role in the development of diabetes, as is genetic pre-disposition. While you may believe that type II diabetes occurs only in overweight people, this is not accurate. About one in eight type II diabetics is of normal weight, and they may suffer from a more aggressive form of the condition. The epigenetic link tying this picture together could be a direct one, in which portions of the genome controlling genes that affect glucose and insulin metabolism are turned off by dietary factors (such as glucose or related molecules) present in high concentrations in the blood of obese people. Or it could be that dietary factors cause obesity and the disruption of metabolism releases molecules that cause the expression of the disease. And of course there are genomic mutations in the DNA which predispose people to diabetes, engaging in back and forth interaction with epigenetic factors.

Sounds pretty complicated, right? How do we separate out the epigenetic contribution from this complex interacting web of causes? Well, it's not easy, but it can be done. That's what we'll address in this chapter.

Diabetes: An Epigenetic Disease?

It would be impossible to prove that diabetes is solely due to epigenetic modifications or intervention, since the complex and varied contributions are interwoven and difficult to separate from one another. However, we can offer a convincing body of observations that I believe will establish epigenetic modifications of the genome as a major contributor to diabetes.

Returning to our detective story, let's see how many smoking guns we can accumulate in our arsenal.

Now if diabetes is truly an "epigenetic" disease, then one strong piece of evidence would come from studies of genes known to predispose individuals to diabetes. We would expect that such genes would be epigenetically modified in diabetic experimental animals and in human diabetic subjects. It turns out that this is true.

One of the best examples of a lab animal with a condition very much like the human form of type II diabetes is the "db/db" mouse (Figure 11), which suffers from a mutation in a gene controlling fat metabolism.[4] However, whether the animal actually manifests the diabetic state depends on the rest of his genetic makeup. There are dozens of different lab mouse strains with dissimilar genetic makeup. The db/db mouse will be diabetic in some strains and not in others. This means there is an interaction or cross talk between these many genes, which is exactly what we see in the human disease. So this is a very accurate reflection of the disease as it occurs in ourselves, and gives us a lot of confidence that conclusions we draw from studying these unfortunate creatures will reveal secrets that would be otherwise unknowable.

There are a number of proteins that are known to be critical to the expression of diabetes; two of them are cell surface receptors for insulin and for something called insulin-like growth factor. As we've mentioned before receptors are complex proteins that are fused into the cell membrane and act as gatekeepers, controlling what gets in and out of the cell. Their shape allows them to bind much smaller molecules in a finely

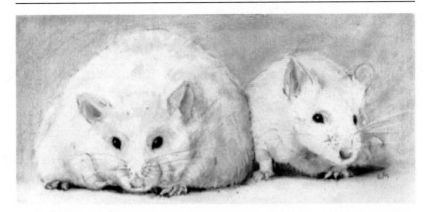

Figure 11. The db/db mouse. Shown is a db/db mouse (left) with normal litter mate that lacks the mutation. The db/db mice are obese, overeaters, cold intolerant, insulin resistant, and infertile. This mutation causes diabetic dyslipidemia, a major factor contributing to the accelerated atherosclerosis in type 2 diabetes mellitus. Within six weeks of age, db/db mice developed significant obesity, fasting hyperglycemia, and hyperinsulinemia. Drawing by Elise Morrow.

crafted, lock and key fashion. Once bound they can move molecules into the cell and release them, so they behave as very specific guardians and porters. They, like all proteins, are coded by genes in the DNA, and they can be epigenetically controlled. That means that they have the CpG sequences in front of them, and these can be methylated, dampening or even shutting off their expression completely.

When the genes for these proteins were studied in the db/db experimental mice, they were methylated and protein production for the insulin-like growth factor receptor was severely depressed. Without the receptor, glucose metabolism is improperly regulated and the animals develop a diabetic condition. So this is a clear example of a diabetic state under epigenetic regulation.

This research supports the epigenetic link, but there are many other studies that approach the question from different points of view, and reach the same overall conclusion. Some studies have now examined the role of DNA methylation in diabetes and its complications.[5] There are many animal studies demonstrating that when promoters are methylated there is a silencing of genes needed for proper pancreatic function, and resulting diabetes.

Take for example a study using diabetic zebrafish, a popular fresh-water aquarium resident. You might be surprised to learn how widely these creatures are employed today in health related research, since unlike mammals, they are a long way from ourselves, in terms of their evolutionary separation. But they are easy and cheap to raise and are said to have a playful disposition. They are also transparent, so one can insert genes into these creatures that code for proteins with fluorescent markers and follow the genes' progress through the animal's body.[6] If cells from the subject have received the gene, one can shine an ultraviolet light and the fluorescent proteins glow dramatically (you can buy them for your home aquarium). Finally, zebrafish possess amazing regenerative powers, and we can perform experiments on them that couldn't be done on other organisms. And in many instances we can generalize a lot from findings made with them.

It turns out that there is a drug, streptozotocin, that damages the pancreas and induces a diabetic-like state, and hyperglycemia (high blood sugar) in zebrafish. This is a hallmark of diabetes, but in the zebrafish, when the drug is removed, the damaged pancreas recovers and the blood glucose levels return to normal. There is another accompanying phenomenon, impaired wound healing, that occurs in the streptozotocin treated animals. Zebra fish are spectacularly adept at wound repair, much more than mammals, and this function is interrupted by the streptozotocin treatment.[7]

There are at the same time dramatic changes in methylation patterns which take place in their DNA. After the drug is removed and the pancreas regenerates, the methylation patterns do not return to normal, even though the blood levels of insulin do. These methylation patterns (hypomethylation of the CpG islands) are passed on to the offspring of the treated zebrafish, and these offspring also suffer from ineffective wound repair. This phenomenon is called metabolic memory, and we see something very similar in human diabetics; when their blood sugar levels are returned to normal, the epigenetic changes and the damage to the tissues are perpetuated. Similar observations have been made in a diabetic rat model. There are some studies that suggest that diabetes can be passed on epigenetically to one's offspring, but there is evidence to the contrary and the question is unresolved.[8]

There's another, quite different way to get at the question in humans. We know that in both human and lab animal tests, dietary restriction can cause epigenetic changes. The availability of vitamins, metals, polyphenols and other molecules can increase or decrease DNA methylation and other epigenetic effects on genes. The results of experiments on animals show that dietary restriction without malnutrition can have beneficial effects and prolong lifespan. The effects are pretty dramatic, but the idea has never caught on with people, and the few studies that have been done gave conflicting results, showing benefits and detriments.[9] In these experiments, age-related diseases including diabetes, cancer, cardiovascular disease, and brain atrophy were substantially decreased. On the other hand, severe dietary restriction to the point of malnutrition can have the opposite effect; it can result in a shortened lifespan and exacerbate disease conditions. In both situations changes in methylation patterns and other epigenetic factors are seen, but the changes are quite different in the two situations.

These observations are exactly what we would predict if the hypothesis of a role for epigenetic control of the diabetic state were correct. So perhaps we have a nice smoking gun, but it's not clear in what direction it is pointed, because a lot of the details remain to be filled into our story. Scientists are uncomfortable with models that leave a lot of unresolved questions. These are gradually being addressed, but epigenetics is a complex science, and it will take years or decades before we completely understand the relationships between genetics, epigenetics and the environmental contributions to diabetes.

Perhaps one of the most powerful research studies that supports an epigenetic basis for diabetes comes from work done by Dr. Margaret Morris, a scientist at the University of New South Wales in Australia. She studied rats made obese by feeding them a special very high caloric diet. She was then able to separate out the epigenetic influence on diabetes from genetic and environmental contributions by observing the offspring of the obese males. Since the males contribute only their sperm to the next generation, this eliminates the effect that an obese female's intrauterine environment might have on the development of the offspring. It also separates out genomic mutations, since the parental rats were raised on a diet that caused them to become obese, thus the weight gain had to be an environmental or epigenetic effect. There is no evidence whatsoever that diet caused mutations in the DNA code that would be detectable in the offspring.

Morris and her collaborators found that the male rats' offspring displayed increased body weight, and impaired glucose tolerance and insulin sensitivity, hallmarks of a pre-diabetic state. Moreover, genes involved in diabetes were hypomethylated in both the fathers and their offspring. This work was the first demonstration of an epigenetic effect on the genome caused by a high fat diet and passed on to the next generation.[10]

There is an historical event that is of particular relevance to our epigenetic smoking gun argument; that is the terrible "famine winter" of 1944–45 in Holland.[11] At that point World War II was moving to its final conclusion. Southern Holland had been liberated by the Allies, but in their rush to Berlin, the Allies left the north and western provinces in the hands of the Germans. As an act of reprisal against the civilian population, the Germans cut off food supplies and for a very discrete period of seven months, Dutch citizens struggled to survive on a daily intake that shrunk to approximately 400 calories. Their plight was so dire that they were reduced to eating tulip bulbs and virtually anything they could obtain to sustain themselves from day to day. During this period, registries and health care remained intact, so that individuals who were prenatally exposed to this famine can be traced. Moreover, the period of famine was clearly defined, and official food rations were documented. Over the years the health status of the survivors and their children has been followed, and in 2008 the methylation status of the insulin-like growth factor II gene in individuals conceived during the famine and matched controls (people born during this period in parts of the country not occupied by the Germans, who were able to obtain adequate nutrition) was studied. This gene has been shown to be under epigenetic control, and animal studies have shown that early embryonic development is crucial for establishing a normal pattern of gene expression.

The striking finding was that after six decades, the IGF-II gene was less methylated in the exposed population than in the matched controls. This pattern is a predictor of diabetes and pre-diabetic states in later life. And to add to the load of evidence, there is increased DNA methylation of a group of genes that make RNA molecules that carry out gene regulation of genes regulating glucose tolerance, an important component of the diabetic picture.

Even more astonishing is the fact that when the children of the women who were pregnant during the famine grew up and had children of their own they were *also* smaller than average. These observations argue that the famine experienced by the mothers caused epigenetic alterations that were passed down to the next generation.

I must add a cautionary note. In discussion with Dr. Shuk-Mei Ho, a professor at the University of Cincinnati, she admonished that there have been other studies on human famine victims in Shanghai and Leningrad during World War II, and the outcome of these studies was somewhat different from those associated with the Dutch Famine Winter of 1944–45. In addition there is much less documentation and followup on these events, so it is difficult to compare them with Dutch famine. There are also ongoing studies of Swedish famines that occurred during the 19th century.[12]

The fact that the children and grandchildren of victims showed epigenetic changes is highly significant, but it does not prove that epigenes were actually transmitted through changes to the epigenome. But the critical test, in terms of epigenetic transmission, would be the fourth generation.

Dr. Ho explained, "Since the woman's uterine environment was modified by the starvation regime, one could argue that the transmission was through a modified intrauterine environment, rather than through the epigenome. And since a developing female fetus already has formed the eggs that will constitute the third generation, they too could be modified by the starvation conditions that the grandmother was subjected to. However, if the great grandchildren of the women who underwent starvation show these changes, then that proves that at least some epigenetic traits can be passed through the germ lines of eggs and sperm."

You can see that as our understanding of epigenetics and its implications grow, the fragility of our hereditary endowment becomes more and more evident. We now know that even physical exercise can bring about modification of the histone proteins, the gene modulators known to be important in epigenetic control. Now studies on human skeletal muscle subjected to exercise regimes demonstrate a number of genes controlling the production of enzyme involved in glucose metabolism.[13]

Collectively, these studies make a strong case for a role of epigenetics in the development of diabetes in both experimental animals and in humans. There's much more to do before the picture is filled in, but we have the outlines of an understanding of the relationship between epigenetics and diabetes. Perhaps the most critical question is whether human contributions to environmental pollution are responsible for the increase we see in the frequency of this condition.

Environmental Epimutagens and Diabetes: What's the Evidence?

If diabetes is linked to epigenetic causes, and if exposure to epimutagenic chemicals and other substances in the environment is increasing, we would expect to see the overall rate of diabetes increasing. This is exactly what we see in studies conducted all over the world. In 1995 the incidence of diabetes, both type I and type II was 4.5 percent but by 2010 it had risen to 8.2 percent. Many studies from different countries have produced similar findings. Of course this does not prove that this increase is due to epigenetic factors; there could be many other causes, and simply because two things occur simultaneously this does not prove that one is the cause of the other.[14]

We certainly know that the level of chemicals in the environment and in our bodies which are thought to be epimutagens is increasing. Studies on the Old Order Mennonites, who, because of their conservative rural life style are less exposed to these compounds, have been found to have lower concentration in their urine. This is hardly surprising, since BPA (Bisphenol A, the widely used plastics additive) and related compounds are present in many cosmetics and household products, which the Mennonites, because of their religious beliefs, refrain from using.[15]

We know that type II diabetes is highly correlated with obesity, and that obesity has increased dramatically in many parts of the world in recent decades. So it could be that obesity causes diabetes, but not through epigenetic mechanisms. Perhaps it causes physiologic changes that disrupt the individual's metabolism and destroy the insulin-producing pancreatic cells. Or it could be that obesity causes epigenetic changes in the genome either directly or indirectly in the manner that I outlined earlier in this chapter. Or it could be that a number of different mechanisms are at work here, and they feed off of one another. We will need more evidence before we can argue a cause and effect relationship. So let's examine some specific situations.

For the last decade a research group in France has carried out studies on the effects of maternal obesity on metabolic disturbances in the children of such mothers. Evidence from both human and animal studies indicate that obesity triggers alterations in fetal development through epigenetic programming. These induce long-term change in gene expression resulting in cardiovascular disease and diabetes in the children in later life. The authors of these studies suggest metabolic products attach to the specific genes in the DNA, driving epigenetic effects with serious consequences.

What if we could see the effect of increasing doses of epimutagens on lab animals or on human populations? Of course we can't willfully expose humans to these substances, but it turns out that there are situation in which both experimental animals and human subjects have been exposed to chemicals known to be epimutagenic. And what was the outcome?

Studies carried by a group of researchers in China involved the exposure of rat pancreatic cells to low levels of bisphenol A and endocrine disruptors. Endocrine disruptors are a class of compounds with significant epigenetic effects. They interfere with normal hormone function. Hormones are chemical messengers; we're all well aware of their effects on our reproductive behavior and how their ascendance at puberty can change loveable cherubic children into rampaging pathological teenagers. These are the steroid hormones, relatively simple chemical molecules that combine with cell proteins called receptors and internalize in the cell, sitting on the DNA, and activating genes. You can appreciate what an amazing and sensitive system of control this is; hormones activate an enormous range of physiological systems and functions. Much of the activation is mediated through epigenetic signals, in which the hormone activates methylation patterns. The steroid hormones have been around in many permutations for eons; this is the reason that hormones act as universal signals across the animal and plant kingdom.

The amounts of the compounds were equivalent to levels that are found in the environment and both are known to be epimutagenic. The changes they caused in the pancreatic cells were significant and caused impairment of their insulin secretion ability. This resulted in glucose and insulin intolerance and progressive damage to the insulin-producing cells of the pancreas.[16]

When mice were given short-term treatments of low doses of BPA their metabolism was slowed and insulin signaling was disrupted in peripheral tissues. These are precisely the features of a pre-diabetic condition in humans.

One of the most important research tools for investigating epigenetic influences is another experimental mouse carrying a gene mutation called agouti Avy. These mice can vary in color from brown to yellow, depending on their genetic background and their diet. The more yellow the coat color of the mice, the more they tend toward obesity and type II diabetes. When pregnant females carrying embryos with the agouti gene are fed BPA in their diets, there is a significant shift toward a greater number of yellow, obese and diabetic offspring.[17]

A large study of U.S. adults, the National Health and Nutrition Examination Survey (NHANES), found that greater than 93 percent of those assessed had detectable levels of BPA in their urine. Because many health related measurement of the participants were measured it was possible to show that there was a significant positive association between peripheral arterial disease and BPA levels in the urine of the participants. Peripheral arterial disease is a important form of cardiovascular disease, and is closely related to diabetes risk. These studies are ongoing, so we can expect that they will be added to in the near future.[18]

There are also studies in humans that are inconclusive. Recently, a Korean research team looked at a large number of people included in a national biomonitoring survey, comparing diabetes and non-diabetes for their levels of BPA in their circulation. While the diabetic individuals had slightly higher levels of BPA, the difference was not statistically significant. The authors of this report do not draw conclusions, stating that their finding neither prove nor disprove a link between BPA exposure and diabetes.[19]

Diabetes and Epigenetics: What Can We Conclude?

Given these limitations of the information presently available, I believe that we can draw some firm conclusions. First of all, the evidence that epigenetics place a role in the development of diabetes is "robust," as scientists love to say. That is, it is sturdy, strong or vigorous. This means that while we accept the fact that other factors play a role in its expression, proper epigenetic regulation and control is a necessary component for the expression of this disease; necessary but perhaps not sufficient.

If we accept this statement, then the next and most obvious question concerns the role of the environment. I use the term in its broadest sense, to include diet, drugs, chemicals in our food and surroundings, our fetal environment and even our psychological milieu.

The role of endocrine disrupting chemicals in causing epigenetic damage to humans is a topic of very hot debate (see Chapter 12). Many epidemiological studies show that environmental exposure to these substances is associated with a wide variety of human diseases and disabilities. The European Union, Canada, and recently the United States have banned the use of BPA (probably the most widely disseminated endocrine disruptor) in baby bottles, but the U.S. still allows its use in cans of infant formula, food and beverages. The U.S. Food and Drug Administration website states, "The FDA is supporting reasonable steps to reduce human exposure to BPA, including actions by industry and recommendations to consumers on food preparation." The prestigious Endocrine Society of America has urged a precautionary approach to the regulation of BPA, stating that there is "growing evidence that the chemical has negative health effects as an endocrine disrupting chemical (EDC). Specifically, BPA has been linked to reproductive anomalies, diabetes, and the development of cancer."[20]

In discussing these questions with scientists working in the area of endocrine disruptors, they have stressed to me that more research is needed. BPA has a very short half life (the time it takes half of the compound to break down in the body), so studies done on populations of people in which their BPA levels are correlated with their health status may not be meaningful, especially since it may require years for damage caused by these compounds to accumulate. One of the researchers that I spoke to (who did not wish their name to be used) stated that it will be necessary to carry out longitudinal studies. These are very long-term, time consuming studies in which individuals are followed over periods of years, and both their BPA levels and their health status are followed. And they are expensive, this in a time when federal funding for health research is being drastically cut.

We cannot at this point say how many cases of diabetes are caused every year in our country by exposure to environmental epimutagens. But it would be foolish in the extreme to ignore this gathering storm of evidence. Now let's look at some diseases of the brain whose origins have defied explanation for years.

Alzheimer's Disease and Epigenetics: Castles in the Sand

The Non-Persistence of Memory

Because digital technology is so ubiquitous in our society, we frequently think of our brains as huge computers, but this analogy is false. Our memories are not permanent, unchangeable bytes, but rather evanescent fragments clutched possibly by individual nerve cells, being constantly washed away and then reconstructed, ever changing, slowly worn away and then rebuilt again, imperfectly. Indeed they are castles in the sand. If you don't believe me, download a movie that you saw 30 or 40 or 50 years ago, and see how your memory of it compares with the actual film, which is unchanging.

For a long time, neuroscientists believed that memories were stored throughout the brain, in millions, or billions of nerve cells. But recent work suggests that individual recollections (such as the face of someone we know) may be stored in much smaller numbers of what they refer to as concept cells. Based on this model, they suggest that interactions between concepts can be achieved through sparse networks, in which small groups of cells interact with other small groups. Such a networking architecture would be much more efficient, and would enable the brain to relate one concept (such as a familiar face) rapidly with another (such as the surroundings of the owner of that face).[1]

Yet imperfect as this information storage system is, it works well enough for most of us. We store the really critical things, in the same manner that our forbears living in caves remembered where the saber-toothed tigers hung out, in the same fashion that the wolf pack knows where the elk hide in the frozen forest. This ruthless pattern of natural selection over millions of years has favored the development of what may be the most complex structure in the universe, the human brain. And in selecting for survival of the most intelligent, many collateral abilities were evolved, even though they have no apparent survival value. We learn and then remember how to carve out incredible feats of creativity, in sports, in the arts, in science, in all manner of pursuits. Opera singers learn an entire opera in a language that they do not speak.[2] Medical students go through memorization marathons, learning all the defining features of our anatomy. We remember joyful and tragic events that lodged in our brains decades earlier. For battle-scarred soldiers, their recall works way too well. As imperfect as our memories are, they comprise a vast store of experience. Over the course of our lives, our memories define us, they make us what we are.

But like all our corporeal parts, our brains can wear away and over time function less and less efficiently. People think of this as "normal aging." It is common for normal healthy individuals to recall items, such as names, with increasing difficulty. Yet the process varies tremendously from individual to individual, and in some cases it can undergo an extremely rapid decline and a catastrophic collapse.

Alzheimer's: A Gathering Storm

There are many sorts of memory loss, some the result of trauma; many are associated with aging, the most prominent being Alzheimer's disease. Half or more of cases of dementia are the result of Alzheimer's disease, which is not part of the normal aging process. Classic Alzheimer's disease is a slowly progressive condition, which worsens over time. Alzheimer's disease can be diagnosed with complete confidence only after death, when microscopic examination of the brain reveals the characteristic plaques and tangles in and around the cells of the brain. There is no cure, but treatments are available which will improve quality of life and lessen the symptoms, at least temporarily. There is an early onset form which has a strong genetic predisposition, and can strike its victims as early as in their 40s. It is the result of DNA genomic mutations in one of at least three genes, and it is especially destructive to families, as it clobbers people at a time in their lives when they are in the midst of building their careers, raising children and caring for older family members. The costs of treating Alzheimer's disease are astronomical, and may run to $100 billion per year for the entire United States, with a worldwide financial cost estimated at a staggering $604 billion.[3] Much of this burden is borne by family members, whose lives may be devastated by stress, financial obligations and emotional pain.

Mortality from Alzheimer's disease has increased dramatically in recent years; the age-adjusted death rate increased by almost 39 percent between 2000 and 2010. It is now the sixth leading cause of death in the United States. If these trends continue, the National Vital Statistics System predicts that annual costs will run to $1 trillion by 2050.[4] During this same period, death from cancer, heart disease and stroke have all declined dramatically. Oddly enough, there are wide variations in age adjusted death rates across the United States going all the way from 10.5 (Hawaii) to 43.6 (Washington). There doesn't appear to be any correlation with income, life styles, urbanization or anything else.

With so much misery and suffering flowing from this condition, it is hardly surprising that right now there is an arms race going on between the drug companies to see who can come up with the first really effective treatment for Alzheimer's. Because the incidence of the disease is skyrocketing, it would be impossible to overstate the repercussions that would spill out from such a finding. An effective treatment would be the most important medical advance of the century. This may explain the high failure rate of new drugs for the treatment of Alzheimer's, as drug companies aggressively push their experimental offerings into higher phases of testing, without solid evidence from early, smaller groups of patients. There are many clinical trials of drugs developed for the treatment of Alzheimer's disease, and although there are no cures, currently available therapies can slow the progress of the disease. These failures have motivated the industry to design trials using individuals at risk for the disease before they show signs of the condition.[5]

The justification for this approach is that by the time patients show signs of memory loss, there may have been irreversible destruction of vital brain tissue. Bear in mind that these treatments do not reverse Alzheimer's disease. In general, once brain cells are damaged or destroyed, they don't reestablish themselves. There are studies in animal models using stem cells that are encouraging, but are very preliminary.[6]

But if you could stop progression in the very early stages, victims could hope for something close to a normal life. The problem with this approach is that clinical trials would have to be extremely long before any benefit could be recognized. And these drugs often have severe side effects, so you could be forcing patients into a treatment that would do little or no good, but would come with considerable baggage. In worst of all possible outcomes, we could wind up with drugs of marginal value, unforeseen side effects and little proven benefit.

For decades there has been an ongoing search for the cause of Alzheimer's disease, and although the question is not resolved, it is generally accepted that the brains in afflicted individuals become clogged up with material referred to as plaques. These plaques are composed of a protein known as the beta-amyloid protein. Most models of the disease cast beta-amyloid in the role of an accumulating substance that forms aggregates, eventually blocking the function of the nerve cells. There are a number of drugs now in development that target beta-amyloid.

The beta-amyloid protein is coded by a gene in our DNA, as is a related protein, tau. The tau protein can form tangles of material inside the cell, whereas the amyloid proteins accumulate outside, in the spaces between the cells. The density and distribution of these defective proteins is a signature feature of the disease. Invariably in the early onset form of the disease they are present in elevated levels. They begin to accumulate in the brains of patients long before the appearance of memory loss and other symptoms.

The problem with this hypothesis is that there are patients and experimental animals with accumulations of the amyloid and tau proteins who do not show the manifestations of the disease. So it could be that the amyloid and tau protein accumulations are a result rather than a cause of the disease, or there may be other complicating factors involved. This could mean that drugs aimed at eliminating the proteins would be ineffective.

In a discussion with Dr. Anand Hindupur, of Meridian Bioscience, Inc., he stated that at this time most researchers in the field agree that although the question is a complex one, the amyloid and tau proteins are the causal agents, rather than a result of the disease. Hopefully, the trials currently underway of drugs that target these proteins will help to resolve this impasse.

Is Alzheimer's Disease Inherited?

Clearly, early onset Alzheimer's is inherited in the same way that blue eyes and brown hair are inherited, by simple alteration in genes, passed to us by our parents. But this is only a small fraction, perhaps 2 percent, of the total cases. Here we're referring to the late onset type of Alzheimer's, which is the type that afflicts the vast majority of patients.

The answer to this question is like so many other topics that we deal with in this book: "Yes, but it's complicated." Using data from the human genome project, scientists have screened the entire genomes of late onset patients, looking for mutations that occur in them, but not in normal people. This is called a GWAS or Genome Wide Association Study.[7] In these studies the investigators are looking small changes in the DNA code, not for epigenetic changes. At least ten genes have been identified so far in which each make a small contribution to the risk of the disease. But the authors of these studies caution that none of these mutations is necessary or sufficient for producing the disease.[8]

You may think that this statement doesn't make much sense. How can you have a gene increasing the risk of something and at the same time not being "necessary and sufficient?" Think about it this way. Say, for example, you were raising crops and you used different genetic strains of corn that gave different yields. Then, say you planted them at the time of a major drought. You would find that the yields were all very poor and you might see no difference at all between the best and the worst strains. So the genes were not permitted by the poor environment to express their full potential. This is what we are facing with Alzheimer's disease. Sure, the genetic background is important, but there are other factors, including environment and epigenetic contributions, that interact with it.

Environmental Factors

There are a number of non-genetic players that increase the risk of late adult onset Alzheimer's. These include depression, hypertension, stroke, diabetes, high cholesterol, being overweight, and smoking. Head trauma, a topic much in the news, is also a risk factor. Whereas the association of sports-related head injuries with Parkinson's disease is well-known, the connection to Alzheimer's has not received as much attention. But studies on boxers and former boxers as far back as the 1970s identified repeated head trauma as an important risk factor.[9]

Not everyone who suffers repeated head trauma will develop Alzheimer's; as we noted there are many other risk factors, including the genetic makeup of the individual and other environmental and epigenetic input which influences his sensitivity.

It would be a vast understatement to say that calls to modify the rules of football and boxing in order to limit the risk of head trauma have not been especially popular. Whereas initially the NFL denied a relationship between sports injuries and neurological disorders, the evidence is now so overwhelming that they have agreed to help fund research into the basis of these injuries. A study of almost 3,500 former pro football players found that they were four times as likely to die from Alzheimer's, Parkinson's and Lou Gehrig's disease than members of the general population. The New York Times stated, "America (may) be ready for some football, but the human brain may never be."[10]

As we learn more and more about the biology of brain trauma, there are increasingly calls for the banning of boxing.[11] This may be unnecessary, given the declining popularity of the sport. It is highly unlikely that boxing rules could be changed sufficiently to eliminate the risk, especially in long-term boxers. Obviously, the same is true for football, the most popular sport in America today. The rules have evolved into what they are today because of the demands of television audiences, and it is unlikely that the rules can be changed without totally altering the sport.

We'll have more to say about this problem later on, but changing deeply entrenched patterns of behavior is never an easy task. Think about how long it has taken to modify the public's opinion regarding cigarette smoking. That doesn't mean it can't be done, it just means that it's not easy. There is a large segment of the public that views such efforts as an unpatriotic governmental intrusion of the dreaded nanny state into areas where they have no business meddling. But then, that was the same argument used 50 years ago in the smoking debate.

From an opposite point of view, there are a variety of factors that lower the risk of Alzheimer's, including physical activity, social engagement, mental activity, Mediterranean diets,[12] moderate alcohol and moderate coffee consumption. All of these are pretty enjoyable activities so why should anybody be opposed to them?

You might wonder if cholesterol-lowering drugs like Lipitor would lower your risk of Alzheimer's. Naturally, big pharma would be ecstatic if this were the case. There have been a number of trials to try and find an answer to this question. So far the findings are ambivalent; some positive, some negative, some no response. So there is certainly no consensus on this issue. The FDA is a long way from approving statins or other anti-cholesterol agents for any purpose other than avoiding cardiovascular disease.

Alzheimer's: The Epigenetic Connection

When we talk about epigenetics and the brain, we must consider a lot of evidence that normal memory processing involves epigenetic activation of various genes. In a recent paper[13] the authors argue that the tightly controlled events that occur when memories are processed in the brain are controlled by epigenetically-responsive genes. The studies involve training lab animals to avoid painful experiences, and then analyzing changes in methylation activities in the brain.

These observations may be related to the dysfunction that occurs in Alzheimer's, based on human studies, animal models and from work with cells grown in the laboratory. The same sorts of epigenetic modification to the DNA that we spoke of earlier have been identified in the brain cells of Alzheimer patients on autopsy. Genes that produce enzymes that modify the amyloid and tau proteins are epigenetically modified in the brains of Alzheimer's patients. In a number of tissue culture studies, the cells were treated with chemicals that cause hypomethylation, removing the chemical groups that silence genes. This caused the genes that code for amyloid producing enzymes to be activated, and the amount of amyloid protein in the cells was increased.

There's also research linking Alzheimer's to epigenetic changes brought about by environmental toxins, particularly heavy metals. These

101

include arsenic, nickel, chromium, cadmium, aluminum[14] and especially lead.[15] When cell cultures are treated with these substances there are many changes to the DNA consistent with epigenetic modifications. In particular, individuals exposed to high levels of lead had higher rates of methylation of promoter genes, which could be responsible for the profound disruption of normal metabolism and development. This is an area that cries out for extensive additional research.

Research in the area of Alzheimer's disease and epigenetics is especially difficult, since the critical diagnosis can only be made from brain tissue samples, analyzed at autopsy. There is a lot of research in progress to find reliable markers that could be present in blood samples, but the availability of unambiguous markers is still in the future.

Another problem that we return to repeatedly is the fact that embryos are especially sensitive to environmental damage. It could be that adult nervous systems are more resistant, so ideally the studies would involve sampling exposure to lead and other possibly epigenetically damaging chemicals throughout the lifetime of the subjects, and in pregnant women. But for human studies this would take years, and not many scientists are interested in research projects that will have to be completed by their grandchildren.

Nonetheless, there are still numerous studies that argue for an epigenetic contribution to Alzheimer's. We don't want to say an epigenetic cause, because we've already observed that there are numerous factors that contribute to the final outcome. When investigators have compared both methylation (adding methyl groups to the DNA) of the entire genome and specific regions within the brain cells of postmortem victims of Alzheimer's and compared them with matched controls from the brains of people who died from other causes, they found the typical epigenetic modifications that contributed to the progress of the Alzheimer condition.[16] Some of the genes were over methylated, some were under methylated. Although such studies are laborious, they contribute to our overall understanding of the origins of Alzheimer's disease, and they suggest possible molecules that could be targeted with drugs.

Another study compared autopsy brain tissue of the frontal cortex (the seat of most higher functions and understanding) from matched pairs of individuals with and without Alzheimer's disease.[17] This is very important, as the amount of methylation changes as we age, and it is important to correct for that fact. In addition, different parts of the brain behave differently. This is precisely what we would expect if methylation were important in controlling thought processes. The scientists used a technique that allowed them to examine a very large number of places in the genome where methylation could occur, including the so-called CpG islands, and other sites containing stretches of CpG. They found at least 26 of these regions that differed between the brain tissues of people with and without Alzheimer's. Some were under methylated and some were over methylated, meaning that in some cases genes were turned on, making more of their products, and in other instances the genes were ramped down, making less.

Epigenetic-Based Therapies

If Alzheimer's has (at least in part) an epigenetic basis, then it should respond to drugs that target epigenetic processes, in the same manner that some success in treating the epigenetic basis of cancer has been obtained. Considering two types of epigenetic modifications, changes to the core histones and modification of the cytosine molecules of the DNA, we can inquire whether chemical interruption of these processes could play a role in memory, and if so, could the destruction of memory in the course of Alzheimer's be interrupted?[18]

The answer appears to be yes. When mice are trained to perform certain tasks, and treated with a compound that inhibits the enzyme histone deacetylase, they formed more connections in the brain and their memories of a particular fear response improved.

It is becoming evident that Alzheimer's and other brain disorders are associated with improper balances within histone acetylation mechanisms.[19] Drugs developed from histone deacetylase inhibitors have emerged as potential new strategies for battling neurodegenerative disease. These molecules enhance performance of the nerve cells, learning and memory in Alzheimer's as well as Huntington's disease and Parkinson's disease. Scientists are looking at a variety of cell culture models and in vivo mouse models of neurodegenerative diseases, and the potential application of HDAC inhibitors to prevent and treat these disorders.

103

Another approach is through DNA methylation. We have considered this phenomenon on many occasions in the book, as one of the major modes of genetic regulation. It was once believed that this was a relatively fixed process: "what you see is what you get." Now we know that it's not static at all, and can switch back and forth with relative ease. So this means genes could be turned on and off over and over again through this process. When rats were taught a particular fear response, the methylase enzymes were cranked up in the part of the brain associated with learning the response (known as the forebrain), and this hypermethylation persisted for weeks.

A number of studies give evidence that histone deacetylase reduces the histone acetylation of genes important for learning and memory. This phenomenon, observed in Alzheimer's patients, is potentially reversible with drugs that inhibit the histone deacetylases.[20]

But, it's important to keep in mind that these studies are preliminary, and years of laboratory work and clinical trials will be required before drugs based on this approach are approved by the FDA.

Why Has the Incidence of Alzheimer's Disease Increased So Dramatically?

One hundred years ago, Alzheimer's disease was virtually unknown in the United States and this is still the case in the underdeveloped world.[21] By and large, Alzheimer's is an affliction of industrialized countries. This suggests that there is something special in our environment which is ramping up its incidence. However, it cannot be industrialization per se, since Japan's rate is one tenth that of the U.S. and Germany's (much more industrialized than the U.S.) only one fifth. There are so many differences in the manner in which these societies are structured that it is not possible to sort them out presently.[22]

I cited statistics documenting the astonishing increase in the incidence of Alzheimer's earlier in this chapter, including the suggestion that heavy metal toxicity may be responsible. Dr. George Brewer[23] of the University of Michigan argues that copper toxicity may be the fundamental cause of this increase. He hypothesizes that copper plumbing, excessive meat consumption and dietary supplements containing copper may be responsible. Vitamin supplements containing copper are widely used throughout the U.S., even though there is no evidence that copper deficiency is rampant in our country.

Excess copper, introduced into our bodies by whatever means, could act to cause epigenetic modification by inducing or shutting down enzymes that are part of the epigenetic program, such as demethylases or histone deacetylases.

While this is an interesting concept, the evidence for it is circumstantial and there could be many other factors in our industrialized environment that act through epigenetic or other mechanisms to drive up the incidence of Alzheimer's. These questions cry out for answers, but this may require a whole new mobilization of our research community.

A Vaccine for Alzheimer's?

Despite a mind-boggling array of high tech medicine that dominates our current approach to dealing with illness, there is no drug or remedy or therapy that works as well as vaccination. This approach to treating disease goes back at least to the 18th century, when crude vaccines against smallpox were developed. One of the greatest medical triumphs of the 20th century was the elimination of polio through the polio vaccine. Mobilizing the body's own superb protective mechanisms can prevent a whole litany of terrible sicknesses at virtually no cost, whereas curing people once they get sick is often beyond the reach of anything that medical science has to offer, no matter how high tech or costly.

Do Vaccines cause diseases such as autism? Absolutely not. This point has been investigated over and over and over again, and there has never been a reliable, solid study that supports this contention. There are, however, innumerable studies that have found no link between vaccination and autism.[24] This very dead horse has been beaten to death over and over again. We need to give it a proper burial and move on.

It will come as no surprise that there are many scientific teams that are struggling to develop an effective vaccine against Alzheimer's disease. Studies with animal models and even human trials have produced encouraging results. In a mouse model, vaccination with a portion of the amyloid protein molecule prevented the development of the characteristic plaques, and in older mice it significantly reduced them. Vaccination reduced age-dependent learning deficits, which correlated with reductions in both soluble amyloid and tau proteins.

These exciting results encouraged a clinical trial which unfortunately was halted prematurely, as 6 percent of the patients who had received the vaccine developed meningoencephalitis (an extremely serious inflammation of the coverings of the brain). But in the same trial, some of the patients showed marked decrease in the loss of their intellectual functions. These trials are now being repeated using a design which will hopefully retain the efficacy of the vaccine while at the same time protecting the patients from their own inflammatory reactions.[25]

Back to the Future

In the century since the psychiatrist and neuropathologist Alois Alzheimer first commented on the disease that came to bear his name, much has been learned, yet there is still a long road to travel. It is probable that Alzheimer's disease will be found to have multiple causes, in the same way that we recognize that cancer is a family of diseases, with a variety of causes, and fortunately, a range of treatment options. Indeed, an understanding of the epigenetic connection to memory opens the door to treatment options that could alleviate diseases of the mind, or augment normal intellectual processes so as to improve our mental capacities.

Finally, can we conclude that environmental chemicals known to cause epigenetic changes and damage could play a role in the increases we seen in the recent years in the frequency of Alzheimer's? The answer to this question is part of our broader understanding of the role of epigenetics in health and disease.

8

A Basket of
Mental Disorders

Major Psychoses Are Linked to Epigenetics

I have argued in preceding chapters that many diseases are linked to epigenetic modifications. This means that the genome, epigenome and the environment are all contributing to the overall picture or phenotype of the individual. This is a difficult concept, and it is not intuitively obvious in the fashion that, for instance, we recognize hemophilia to be the due to a gene mutation. It's been known for a long time that on the X chromosome there is a stretch of DNA with a lot of bases that specify one of the proteins that causes the blood to clot. In this case we can say that if a person has an alteration in the critical region of that gene, he will make a defective protein that will not clot appropriately. He or she will surely have hemophilia. If not, no hemophilia.[1] This concept is so simple and straightforward that it can be taught in grade school. But I don't believe that any grade schools are teaching epigenetics these days, even in Lake Woebegone.

If our inheritance is dictated by a complex dance between these three forces, and if we're talking about such obscure terms as the "architecture" of genetic structures, then perhaps we can begin to understand why such a bewildering collection of diseases and conditions are influenced by the epigenome. Let's consider two well-known and widespread conditions, and see what are their possible epigenetic connections.

Schizophrenia

We know that a wide range of mental disorders have at least in part a genetic basis, because many, many twin studies carried out over the years have shown that identical twin pairs are more concordant for these conditions than are fraternal twin pairs. Earlier I pointed out the flaws in the twin study method and the fact that twin studies at their best, provide only a tentative conclusion that the trait has some inherited basis. Many of these studies were done years before the role of epigenetics in complex mental maladies was appreciated. In retrospect it is hardly surprising that twin studies were hard to interpret and did not establish the existence of specific genes for these conditions. If genes responsible for mental disorders can be turned on and off by epigenetic modification, perhaps brought on by environmental actors, then this would tend to make identical twin pairs less concordant for mental diseases, causing the investigators to attribute this variability to environmental factors, and they would be correct. But this means that we cannot put heredity and environment into neat little boxes, the way the eugenics movement attempted to do in the 20th century.[2]

Schizophrenia and bipolar disorder are chronic, frequently occurring conditions. Schizophrenia is characterized by a wide range of abnormalities in perceptual, emotional, cognitive, and motor processes including delusions and abnormal thought patterns that cluster in three categories[3]: first, positive symptoms which include delusions, perceptual disturbances and hallucinations, and abnormalities in thought patterns; secondly, negative symptoms which include asociality, avolition (impaired initiative, motivation and decision making), mood disturbances, alogia (a paucity in the amount or content of speech), and anhedonia (reduced capacity to experience pleasure) and finally, cognitive abnormalities such as impairment of memory and selective attention.

Bipolar Disorder

Bipolar disorder is a mood disorder characterized by episodes of mania (extremely elevated mood, energy, unusual thought patterns, and sometimes psychosis) and depression. Schizophrenia and bipolar disorder each affect about 1 percent of the world's population and cause great distress to affected individuals, emotional burden to their families, and social disruption. Both the quality and quantity of life are severely affected. Not surprisingly, suicide rates are greatly elevated over the frequency within the general population, and medical complications lower lifespan.

The average life expectancy of patients with schizophrenia and bipolar disorder is 56.3 years. These disorders are thought to be due to abnormalities involving the development of the brain leading to disruptions in its neural circuitry.[4]

Epigenetic Determination

There are three types of cells in the central nervous system, the neurons that carry the signals and the astrocytes and oligodendrocytes that support the neurons. Think of the astrocytes and oligodendrocytes as the emperor's entourage, making sure he is kept comfortable and that all his needs are fulfilled. All three types come from stem cells, and they are made continually throughout the life of the individual. This a major surprise: when you were growing up no doubt you were taught in high school and college that early in embryonic development you got all the brain cells you were ever going to get, and throughout life the body is constantly eliminating cells. But now we know that epigenetic effects, in concert with cues from the outside is pushing differentiation and determining the fate of these cells throughout life.

This is a very exciting and positive body of work (see, not everything I'm telling you in this book is depressing and gloomy) because it suggests that mental disorders might be reversible if we understood them thoroughly. The epigenetic tools in the box are the usual suspects: methylation, histone modification and microRNA mobilization and expression. There is some evidence that all three play a role in normal and abnormal mental states.

For instance, some gene promoters for genes that make important structural proteins in the brain were found to be methylated in the brains of dead individuals who were patients with schizophrenia and bipolar disorder.

Neurotransmitters are chemicals in the brain that are important in moving signals from one neuron to another. They play a role in many neurological diseases. And in at least one case, the genes for enzymes that metabolize these neurotransmitters have been found to be abnormally methylated.

Histone modifications have been proposed as contributing to the pathogenesis of dysfunction in the brains of schizophrenics. It has been reported that enzymes known as deacetylases (important in histone modification and the remodeling of the chromatin) are increased in the prefrontal areas of the brains of schizophrenics.

In the case of bipolar disorder, a number of gene specific methylation changes have been noted in tissue from the frontal cortex of post-mortem patients. In the area of microRNAs, differences in miRNA in patients as compared to controls were observed. There are also abnormalities in miRNAs from post mortem analysis.[5]

So there's a lot of tantalizing information implicating epigenetic mechanisms in major psychotic diseases. But it will take additional data to build a really conclusive, detailed picture of the relationships between epigenetic mechanisms and these diseases.[6]

Schizophrenia and Bipolar Disorder Are Increasing in Frequency

Numerous studies demonstrate that the incidence of schizophrenia and bipolar disorder is increasing. This belief is based on a number of factors: the increasing number of severely mentally ill among homeless and incarcerated individuals; reports that at least one-third of the approximately 600,000 homeless individuals have a severe psychiatric disorder; a Department of Justice study stating that 16 percent of inmates in local jails and state prisons have been treated for psychiatric disorders. Summarizing, Torrey states, "We are left with an epidemic of schizophrenia and bipolar disorder that presently affects 4 million Americans, that slowly kills by suicide 15 percent of those afflicted and that costs the nation over $110 billion each year in direct and indirect costs, an invisible plague that increased as much as 10-fold over the last century and that appears to still be increasing."

Psychiatric Disorders and Drugs

It turns out that many psychiatric disorders are linked to epigenetics mechanisms, including depression. This condition, including its more severe manifestation, major depressive disorder, has a lifetime risk of 10–15 percent for the U.S. general population, is associated with excessive sadness, and a range of negative symptoms including changes in sleep pattern and appetite. Drugs used to treat depression such as valproate cause epigenetic changes in experimental animals and interfere with histone methylation.[7] There are three categories of epigenetic drugs that are being actively investigated for their ability to treat psychosis: drugs inhibiting histone deacetylation; drugs decreasing DNA methylation; and drugs targeting microRNAs, so this covers the major drivers of epigenetic actions that we have discussed previously.

Environmental Contributions

There is a substantial research into the question of environmental contributions to major psychoses through the epigenetic route, as we have touched previously. Such forces that could modify the epigenome include childhood adversity, migration, urban residence, nutrition and advanced paternal age. Earlier in this book we talked about the Dutch hunger winter and how the starvation conditions could have resulted in epigenetic-based changes to children conceived during this period. In fact, the incidence of schizophrenia in sons conceived during this period was twice that of matched controls.[8] It has been suggested that conditions that disrupt normal metabolism could affect methylation patterns in the DNA of these children, leading to an increase in the incidence of schizophrenia.[9] There has been an independent confirmation of these studies from the Chinese famine that offspring of prenatally nutritionally compromised mothers had a higher risk of schizophrenia.[10]

A War Within

For centuries psychiatric conditions were considered to be the work of angry gods, witches or demons.[11] For the early part the 20th century they were thought to be due to bad parenting, unresolved Freudian conflicts, or innate failure on the part of the individual. The eugenics movement of the first half of the 20th century laid the blame on bad genes, and decreed that the problem could be eliminated through sterilization or if that didn't work, more draconian methods. There was no knowledge of their biochemical basis. As information accumulated, their interpretation became more sophisticated, but still lacking in structure or fundamental understanding. Twin studies indicated some genetic contribution, but the exact mechanism was unclear. It is now evident that epigenetic changes are a major contributor to psychiatric disease, and the interaction of the genome and epigenome and the environment are working together to produce the interactions that we see in so many other diseases considered in this book.

The role of environmental factors is increasingly recognized as pivotal in the development of these conditions. Epigenetics now provides specific mechanisms by which neuroregulatory proteins are controlled. This allows the development of very detailed and critical models in which the environment drives epigenetic changes affecting output of gene products within the nervous system. So these hypotheses make very specific predictions that can be tested and will allow the development of solid theories of mental function.

Given that epigenetically driven diseases are potentially reversible, there has been much interest focused on drugs that influence these molecular changes. The author of a recent review points out that none of these drugs is specific for the genes that are epigenetically modified, therefore side effects could be unacceptable, and much clinical testing will be required before patients can be routinely treated with these substances.[12]

9

Epigenetics and Autism: The Queen of the Night

A Condition Without a Clear Description

What would you do if you were trying to raise a child with a strange malady, for which there were no cure, no treatment and no notion concerning why your child was cursed with this condition? And say the disease were devastating and raising this child affected your whole family, and you had no idea whether your child would ever improve, or would continue to get sicker and deteriorate? And say that you were bombarded relentlessly with conflicting explanations of the cause of this disorder, and you had little means of verifying or rejecting conflicting information? Chances are you'd be bitter, frustrated and willing to try anything that could favor your child's chances for a better life. And that's exactly the situation in which families with autistic children find themselves.

A condition that manifests itself through impairment of social interactions and by repetitive behavior, autism is perhaps the most prominent mental state to be linked to an epigenetic basis. "Highly variable" and "increasing in frequency" are two phrases most commonly used to describe it. A striking property of these children is their need for certain rituals and events which may be obsessive with sporadic motor activity (such as hand-flapping or head-banging). These patterns of behavior create a tense and difficult environment, and are a major cause of stress for these individuals and their families. Autism appears early in infancy and steadily worsens, yet some individuals can show high functioning performance, whereas other may be severely retarded. The rule is that there are very few rules.

It was only in the 1980s that autism was recognized as having a biological basis, rather than simply resulting from a failure of the parents to raise their children properly. Since then, there have been many anatomical studies that have clearly demonstrated developmental abnormalities, often originating long before birth. In recent years a large body of evidence has determined that environmental, genetic and epigenetic factors all mix together to spawn this condition.

Autism has received so much attention and has become such a hot button of controversy because there are so many unknowns and bitter disagreements revolving around it. While it appears to be inherited, there is no simple genetic pattern, typical of the many complex diseases we have already considered. Although about a third of children are incapable of basic communication, some autistic individuals may develop high levels of performance, while at the same time failing to achieve the level of intuition and social interaction that is so common in most people that it is self assumed.

Some of the characteristic features of autism spectrum disorder include loss of language or social skills, poor eye contact, no smiling or social responsiveness, and later in life, impaired ability to make friends with peers and stereotyped, repetitive, or unusual use of languages.[1]

Perhaps the most critical question revolves around the frequency of autism, which is currently said to be one in 88. Between 2000 and 2008 (the most recent date for which accurate data from the United States are available), the Center for Disease Control reported that the frequency of autism rose at an astronomical pace, from one in 150 children to the accepted figure of one in 88.[2] While changes in the way autism is diagnosed, and heightened concern over infants and children with learning problems may account for some of the upsurge, all of the authorities interviewed for this book were convinced that there has been a real rise in the incidence of autism in recent decades.[3] There have been several well documented studies in peer reviewed journals, and all come to the conclusion that while changes in the criteria for autism diagnosis may account for some of the expansion, it is trivial compared to the vast increases observed during these periods. So we have a very large and unaccountable increase in autism, seen in many countries. There is no possible DNA-based genomic mechanism, such as an accumulation of new mutations in the genome, that could account for such a calamity.[4]

There are some strident objections to the high rate of autism diagnoses. Dr. Allen Francis is professor emeritus and former chair of psy-

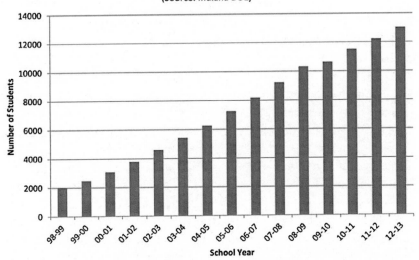

Number of Students Identified with Autism Spectrum
Disorders in Indiana's Public Schools
(Source: Indiana DOE)

Figure 12. Increase in Autism Incidence. Approximately 53 percent of the increase in autism prevalence over time may be explained by changes in diagnosis (26 percent), greater awareness (16 percent), and an increase in parental age (11 percent). While this research is beginning to help us understand the increase in autism prevalence, half of the increase is still unexplained and is not the result of better diagnosis, greater awareness, and social factors alone. This residual increase is attributed to environmental factors interacting with epigenetic and genetic susceptibilities.

In 2009, the Centers for Disease Control issued a report based on a sample of eight year olds, and concluded that the prevalence of autism had risen to one in 110 in American children. By 2012, using a similar sample, it was announced that the incidence had climbed to one in 88. Based on these latest numbers, one in 54 boys and one in 252 girls are being diagnosed with an autism spectrum disorder. From: Increasing Incidence of Autism Spectrum Disorders Continues in Indiana. Contributed by Dr. Cathy Pratt, BCBA-D, Director, Indiana Resource Center for Autism. See http://www.iidc.indiana.edu/?pageId=361%20-%20sthash.FB6Deon7.dpuf#sthash.cvtsb2nY.dpuf. Reprinted with permission from Indiana Resource Center for Autism. Accessed October 10, 2013.

chiatry and behavioral science department at Duke University. In his writings he claims that there cannot possibly be as high rate of autism as reported. He blames this excess on a greedy drug industry that makes money off of overprescribing medication to healthy people.[5] But it would appear that that Francis' opinion is very much a minority view. The vast majority of professionals in the field agree with the conclusion that I have presented here.

What Defines Autism?

If individuals diagnosed as autistic are so heterogeneous, is there a common designation and a collection of common features that we can agree upon? It appears that there is. The average cranial size of autistic children is larger than normal, because their brains are bigger. When the anatomy of their brains is examined, there is an increase in the number of structures known as "neocortical minicolumns."[6] These are tiny arrangements in the brain, small vertical columns of hundreds or thousands of brain cells that organize and move signals and are in some way responsible for the elaborate transmission network that enables thought processes to occur. In a human brain there are about 200 million of them, so you can appreciate its staggering complexity, given that these columns are communicating constantly with one another.

But why would having more minicolumns be bad? Intuitively, it seems that it would provide an advantage. We don't really know the answer, but we do know that our bodies have evolved to an optimal state over millions and millions of years, and in the same fashion that you probably couldn't play the piano better if you had ten fingers on each hand, your brain probably won't function optimally with more structures.

The Unknown City in a Strange Land

Think of the brain as a great unknown city, but not a city like Beijing or New York City or Mexico City with 20 million or so inhabitants. A monster megacity, with billions and billions of inhabitants, communicating and accessing one another, constantly sending messages back and forth, yet completely organized and ordered, so these signals all blend together into a vast, completely coherent tapestry. It's easy to appreciate why this whole edifice is so fragile and easily damaged.

As the embryonic brain develops, it undergoes a process of growth of the nerve cells and elongation of the projections from the cells' bodies known as axons and dendrites. This process is known as arborization, like the branching of a tree, and during this period, much expansion and pruning of these extensions is occurring.

There has been a lot of excitement lately concerning large scale missions to map this massive communications network. Efforts to do this go back a number of years. In 2007 I took part in a journalism tour of universities and high tech companies in Switzerland with an international group of science writers. On a visit to the Technical University of Lausanne (EFPL), we were treated to a three dimensional film depicting what is referred to as the Blue Brain Project, a massive effort by Swiss researchers to map all the connections in the brain and model it on a supercomputer.[7] Once you have your 3-D glasses in place, the film takes you on a microscopic ride through one of the columns (from a rat), all the nerve cells arrayed in blue. Gliding through a darkened forest of long nerve fibers to the strains of "The Blue Danube Waltz" by Johann Strauss, the experience has a captivating science fiction quality to it, quite lovely and exciting. The project was originated by Henry Markram, a brilliant and charismatic scientist, and also a controversial figure who has rubbed many in the field the wrong way.

Part of the reaction against large scale brain mapping projects is from scientists who are troubled by a scientific effort that has an industrial scale quality to it. These were the same criticisms that were leveled at the Human Genome Project. By and large, scientists formulate a hypothesis and then design experiments to confirm or reject it. These folks reject large scale collaborative science as mindless drone work that sucks off resources from really creative science (remember the "night science" that Francois Jacob used to describe his approach?) that can push back frontiers. Other disparagements are the immense cost of the work and the tiny amount of progress so far, a criticism to which Markram would no doubt take exception. Some authorities have argued that the task is simply too difficult and expensive to take on at this time, but it has captured the imagination of some of the smartest neuroscientists in the world.

There are other large scale efforts in the works to map the brain.[8] Recently the Obama administration has proposed a related project, and if it comes into being, the U.S. and European efforts will no doubt be carried out jointly.[9] If the venture is successful (and there is no assurance that it will be) it will represent an enterprise bigger than the Human Genome Project. The human brain is said to have 100 billion cells and trillions of connections to track down, and so far the results are pretty paltry. The work is progressing, but as you can imagine for an effort of this scale, it will be years in the making and cost billions of euros.

If it does succeed, its promoters argue that it could become a powerful tool in understanding and treating autism and many other conditions that bedevil humanity. Presumably, if we could recreate a human brain on a supercomputer, we would grasp the nature of human essence, the existence of the soul and all the qualities of human consciousness. And with it would come a comprehension of all the disorders of the brain.

Autism: The Ghost in the Machine

Essentially researchers are arguing that autism is due to a botched brain developmental engineering program, in which incorrect signals are transmitted that tell the embryonic brain to produce more nerve cells than it should. The result is an individual with a brain that doesn't work exactly the way normal brains do. It is easy to see how this brain, with extra nerve cells and extra connections, might actually perform better at certain tasks, and yet overall might not be as successful as a normal brain in guiding the owner through life. Such an individual could receive conflicting messages from these cells, and fail at extremely complex tasks such as social interactions.

So how does the description I have presented relate to the root causes, the genes, epigenes and environment? The current picture of how genes program the formation of the brain to produce the final finished individual is by activation of signaling molecules. Think of them as busy little administrators, pulling this magnificent structure together. These controller genes are activated at precisely the right moment in embryonic development, in the same way that all the structures of a building must be added in precisely the right sequence. The worker genes are those that specify the molecules that are gene products, programmed by the DNA.

Frequently complex hypotheses described in research papers in academic journals display elaborate wiring diagrams with arrows connecting the various molecules that are given obscure designations of letters and numbers. Usually in the legend of the figure it will say something to the effect of "for the purpose of simplicity, only the most important connections are shown."

There is no way we can further simplify these blueprints for you, but for this discussion, we really don't need to. The numbers, amounts, placement, arrangement and timing of our workers, administrators and construction crew results from controller genes, rolled into action by the epigenetic messages. In some instances of autism, environmental triggers may activate the epigenetic controls during embryonic development. Later in life, different environmental influences could either dampen or exacerbate the autistic condition. By "environment" this could mean chemicals that turn on and off epigenetics switches, so genes are activated or silenced inappropriately. It is easy to imagine that such an exquisite process could fall prey to internal demons. It is also possible to see why the embryonic period is much more sensitive than the adult phase of the individual's lifespan.

If only certain stages in the life of the individual are sensitive to epimutagens, then we can understand why it so difficult to nail down cause and effect relationships, and put our smoking guns in order on the gun rack. The scheme as presented here may make sense, but a sensible idea does not constitute a scientific proof. So what's the evidence that connects epigenetics and autism?

The Genetic Link

Let's take the three contributing determinants of autism one at a time and talk about the evidence for their role in the disease. The first is the genetic contribution: is autism inherited? Well, in some cases it is, in the sense that we think of Mendel's pea plants, and their simple patterns of inheritance of smooth seeds and wrinkled seeds. These are "all or none" traits, you either have them or you don't. That's why Mendel selected them when he started his studies. There are a few, very rare mutations that cause autism in humans that are "all or none" and that have a simple pattern of inheritance. These are mutations that disrupt the messages so dramatically they have a profound effect, bringing about on their own a full-blown autistic state.[10]

But most autistic people fall into a different category. When we study the inheritance of really complicated traits in humans, we find there are many genes that contribute to the phenotype. Autism is complicated by the fact that the majority of genes associated with the disorder are associated with only one specific symptom.[11] This is hardly surprising, since the brain must have thousands of genes required for its construction. So for instance, if you ask about the genetics of intelligence, it's not something that you have or don't have, it is a continuous spectrum from high IQs down to low IQs. This means you need to look at the question in a different light.

The traditional starting point for studying the inheritance of complex traits is the twin study method, which we've already mentioned. When applied to autism we find that the identical twins are much more concordant than the fraternal twins. But the twin studies don't tell how something is inherited; only that genes play some role. The twin study method is a highly controversial approach to understanding how genes and environment make us who we are. The fact that scientists have been arguing over its validity for the last hundred years is hardly ever broached in presentations to a lay audience. This is a terrible tragedy, since so many political decisions have been based on conclusions drawn from it.[12]

There are mathematical equations that allow one to estimate the relative contributions of heredity and environment to one of these complex traits, say 60/40 or 80/20, depending on how the numbers sort out. The trouble is that twin studies make all sorts of assumptions that are shaky at best, and trying to put a hard number on these observations is a risky proposition. The whole scheme rests on the belief that you can divide up heredity and environment into separate boxes and assign a percent contribution to whatever your studying, be it intelligence, musical ability, athletic talent, or a disease condition. But this is no doubt a false proposition, since we've seen that heredity and environment are so tightly intertwined that it is a fool's errand to try and separate them in the way that these mathematical estimates attempt to do. This is probably why twin studies on the genetics of autism come up with numbers that vary all over the map.[13]

I believe that it is most accurate to say that autism is partially determined by variations in a number of genes, and that certain combinations of variant genes constitute a high risk background. Many people may carry some of these variants and be perfectly normal. The birth of an autistic child will occur only if the environment favors the expression of these genes. But this is only a part of the story.

Are there other ways that we can establish the role of genes in autism? Indeed there are; one can use the tools of molecular biology to go on a search for DNA sequences that show up in autistic children. The usual way this is approached is by comparing entire genomes of autistic and non-autistic people and looking for mutations that are more often found in one group but not in the other. Then one would work their way through these possibilities, searching out the genes that code for proteins playing a prominent role in the functions of the brain.

These large scale scans of the genomes of normal and autistic individuals have turned up hundreds of genes that appear to make small contributions to the possibility of an autistic outcome.[14] However, some of these studies are in conflict with one another, and the contribution of many of the genes to the outcome are so small that their identification is very difficult to replicate. On the other hand, many of the genes that determine the major inherited forms of autism have been thoroughly studied, and have been shown to code for important protein that scaffolding and structure of the brain.

So we are left with a residue of many genes that make a contribution to the risk of autism, but their exact nature and what they do is still largely unknown.

The Epigenetic Link

What the evidence that connects epigenetic changes with autism?

We can consider numerous examples that pull together the autism-genetic-epigenetic connection. Recently, scientists have studied a protein, called SHANK, that is important in the formation of the synapses, the connecting points between nerve cells, where the signal jumps from one cell to another. It turns out that mutations in the DNA of this gene have been found in patients with autism spectrum disorder and moreover in a severe genetic abnormality in which a copy of this gene is missing.[15] The absence of one copy of the SHANK gene has devastating repercussions, resulting in a serious form of autism. About 1 percent of individuals with an autism spectrum disorder have an alteration of the SHANK3 gene. Mice that have been genetically engineered to carry similar mutations display autistic-like behavior.

But there is another way in which alterations of the SHANK gene can result in autism. Within it there are several CpG islands that allow its control in an epigenetic manner. When the SHANK gene's CpG islands are highly methylated, the expression of this vital protein is shut off. Moreover, when cell cultures are treated with chemicals that block methylation, the gene is expressed.

There are a number of studies that provide strong links between autism and epigenetics. SHANK is one of the best studied, but all these fall into comparable patterns, building a massive body of evidence, joining epigenetic signals to expression of the disease.

When the brains of autistic individuals who have died from unrelated causes were analyzed, it was found that the histones in the DNA of the nerve cells of the cortex were modified epigenetically in hundred of genetic regions important in nerve cell function. This is precisely what would be predicted, that epigenetic modifications would be observed in cell types critical to brain function and architecture, and that these epigenetic modifications could cause the nerve cells to malfunction and result in autism or related patterns of behavior.

The Environmental Link

I have already argued that a great deal of evidence supports a prominent role for environmental influences on epigenetic expression; what do we mean by this? Environment could be drugs, chemicals, dietary factors, even psychological input, such as stress. We've seen in previous chapters that there is a wealth of evidence linking disease states to epigenetic causes, brought about through environmental interventions. Is this the case for autism?

The hottest autism potato today is probably the row over vaccination and autism, which has been going on for years. This debate has taken on the trappings of a religion. People who are convinced that vaccination is responsible for cases of autism are not swayed by the fact that no one in the scientific community of autism researchers believes in such a connection. One of the leading autism researchers in the country, Dr. Manuel Casanova from the University of Louisville told me recently that there simply was no credible evidence linking autism and vaccination. This conviction is supported by volumes of research results, approaching the question from every conceivable vantage.[16]

At this time there is great bitterness and frustration among the public that no simple silver bullet has surfaced that would spell the end to autism. I believe that this is one of the most powerful forces motivating parents of autistic children to cling to a belief for which there is not a shred of scientific evidence. But today many people reject scientific evidence that conflicts with strongly held beliefs and go for totally nonsensical notions. No amount of argument will change their belief. This is especially tragic, since the relationship between autism and epigenetics is especially well supported by the data. There are many epigenetic risks to our health, and there is much research to support these concerns. So let's look at the best science available linking autism to environmentally driven epigenetic effects.

If we look for possible substances in our environment that could cause epigenetic damage, there is no shortage of bad actors. In recent decades there has been an immense increase in our exposure to pesticides and fungicides, including organophosphates, pyrethroids and organochlorine. Select populations taken from farming communities have exposed groups that are especially at risk for exposure, bringing to mind the elevation in cases of multiple myeloma occurring in farmers and ranchers. Especially disturbing is a study of children born to mothers in the California Central Valley who had been exposed to organochlorine insecticides.[17] The scientists found that women exposed between days 26 and 81 of their pregnancy were almost eight times more likely to give birth to children with autism spectrum disorder than mothers who received the lowest exposure levels.

But it is not only those living in farming environments who may experience high levels of exposure to these agents. Many people, including pregnant women, may be applying pesticides in and around their homes, using insecticidal soaps on pets and spraying gardens and their surroundings with these agents. These compounds are so wide spread that 83 percent of pregnant women had detectable levels in their blood and urine. Rarely did these individuals take steps to protect themselves, such as bathing pets outdoors and cleaning themselves thoroughly after using insecticidal pet shampoos. Today it may be impossible to find populations who are not exposed to detectable levels of these substances, which means it will be even more difficult to establish cause and effect relationships.

The unfortunate truth is that our civilization is awash in thousands of different chemical agents, and new ones are introduced every day. Only a tiny fraction of these compounds have been tested for health effects and those that have been examined have rarely been thoroughly evaluated for epigenetic effects. These include cosmetics, cleaning products, household solvents, food additives, and painting and varnishing materials.[18]

Living in a World of Hazards

The abhorrent picture which is coming together is one of a disease with extremely serious consequences and growing rapidly in frequency. I stated earlier in this chapter that the most recently available numbers for the United States for the incidence of autism put the chances at one in 88 births. More recent studies from other countries throughout the world show a continuing rise. There are a number of population studies in progress, so we should be seeing precise updates of these numbers for the United States in the near future.

In attempting to understand the causes of the alarming increase in autism, we can rule out an increase in mutations in the DNA as a possible source. Everything we know about mutagenesis makes it clear that the huge increases seen in recent decades are so unprecedented that DNA base-pair mutations can be absolved of responsibility. Nor do simple changes in the way autism is diagnosed account for more than a small fraction of the increase.

The best model brings together the two other partners, the environment and the epigenome. There are two ways this interaction might come about. Agents in the environment could directly act on the developing individual, either at the embryonic stages, or later in development. We know of chemical exposures that are responsible for severe birth defects, so there is precedence for this mechanism. The alternative would be that the agents act directly on the epigenetic sites, causing controller genes to regulate development imperfectly. There is a lot of evidence for this mechanism; Dr. Mike Skinner at Washington State University is one of the most widely recognized authorities on the topic of "epimutagenesis." He has published many peer reviewed articles detailing how a litany of chemical agents can cause severe damage through epigenetic mechanisms in lab animals.

It is not possible at this time to assign a single cause for the astonishing rise in autism, and there may not be one. With the genome wrapped around the epigenome and imbedded in the environment, it will be some time before these effects can be sorted out. The sources of this damage are legion, but the fact that these are complex and difficult questions, and that they may have no simple answers, does not mean that in desperation we should refuse to use wisdom and logic to confront them, nor does it mean that we should give ourselves over to quackery and mendacity.

But with such a large number of chemicals in our environment, and with little knowledge of their risk, we are greatly limited in the steps that we can take to protect ourselves. Of course there are obvious precautions that are listed on the bottles of household cleaners and paints and solvents, such as avoiding unnecessary exposure and thoroughly washing. This of course is even more important when the user is pregnant.

Dr. Manuel Casanova and Emily Williams are experts in the field of autism research at the University of Louisville, and I spoke with them in the preparation of this book. They summarize their current views on epigenetics and autism as follows: "Autism may be indicative of how our environment has changed over time: while a portion of the increased diagnostic rates are due to changes in diagnostic criteria, inclusion of milder cases, and greater general awareness, a majority of the increase is still unaccounted for, and therefore autism may be a barometer for the changing molecular climate."[19] But there are steps that we can take to start an attack on this scourge. We'll get to those soon, but let's see what epigenetics has to say about the end of life.

125

Epigenetic Exercise: Just Do It

Taking Control

In these pages we've talked about how the epigenome responds to internal and external signals. Now evidence is coming together showing that we can make conscious decisions to turn on genes through epigenetic activation. All you have to is sign up at your local gym.

We all know that when we exercise, profound things happen to our bodies, and they're all good. Our heart muscle becomes stronger, our cholesterol levels go down, we may lose weight through elimination of fat and by building up muscle mass, our blood pressure drops, and we feel better overall. We've always assumed all these processes are brought about by increasing protein synthesis, enlarging muscles and the other structures needed for improved performance. So how does epigenetics fit into this picture?

Secrets of Sweat

The first question is, what causes these wonderful changes? It is DNA methylation, histone modification and activation of microRNAs. And of course the first place to look is the human skeletal muscle genes. What we find is they respond by hypomethylation of their promoters so a whole family of muscle protein genes swing into action. You see these changes in humans and mice, in cell cultures. Especially prominent are the genes for myosin, the muscle protein.[1]

We don't ordinarily associate exercise with protection from cancer, but now there is evidence that it does occur, and through the epigenetic route. We talked about tumor suppressor genes, and how their promoters can become methylated, so the gene is no longer expressed, and without this level of cellular protections, tumors develop. And when exercise occurs, these tumor suppressor genes become unmethylated and they begin to produce their respective proteins.[2]

There have always been claims that people who exercise live longer.[3] Could this be true and if so, could it come about through an epigenetic route? In our discussion of the aging process we'll introduce you to the telomeres, the ends of chromosomes that form caps that deteriorate with time, causing the cells to become senescent. Proteins that protect the telomeres and stabilize them are induced by epigenetics mechanisms. There are studies, in humans, suggesting that physical exercise induces these proteins through epigenetic mechanisms.[4] It is likely that the induction by exercise of a number of brain-derived growth proteins can promote mental health and resistance to neurological disorders. One of these, BDNF, is thought to contribute to resistance to Alzheimer's, depression, bipolar disorder and attention deficit hyperactivity disorder.

The connection between healthy heart function and exercise is well known, but until recently there was no clear molecular mechanism known by which this process occurred. During periods of exercise the heart muscle increases in size, the so-called "athlete's heart."[5] At this time signaling proteins that mobilize the proteins needed to drive the expansion of the heart tissue are produced, the result of the induction of many different small RNA molecules through epigenetic signals.[6]

One way to study the relationship between epigenetics and exercise is look at "global" changes in methylation patterns in tissue of volunteers before and after embarking on exercise programs. This can be done by studying methylation of many, many sites (hundreds of thousands!) within the genome using technologies that allow you to scan these sites with automated systems. The results of these studies showed that gene expression was altered throughout, but especially in a number of genes that affect fat cell metabolism.[7]

We are now reaching the point where many scientists are recognizing that changes in DNA methylation are the likely biological mechanism behind the beneficial effects of physical activity. The epigenetic connection also goes a long way toward explaining the fact that when dramatic changes in body metabolism come about as a result of exercise, they don't go away after exercise is terminated. That is, if you crank up your metabolism through exercise, it stays cranked up when you're not exercising. This is precisely the way epigenetics works; it may bring about long-term changes in gene expression.

Using What We Know

You probably didn't expect much of a break from doom and gloom, but I indicated at the outset that epigenetics holds a lot of promise in addition to the specters that it raises. And taking advantage of these findings with regard to the epigenetics of exercise is something that we all can do. There is no exotic science or breakthrough drug required, no laundry list of risks to be avoided.

This is not exactly a self help book; these books are very fond of lists. They always have a title like *The Seven Habits of Highly Effective People* or *A Gentle Path Through the Twelve Steps*. Here's one: *Change-ology: Five Steps to Realizing Your Goals and Resolutions*. But I'm going to make it easy. Just one step. While we all know what we need to do, I find it immensely encouraging that we are moving into an era in which we have a solid understanding of how exercise works.

And this means that shortly we will be able to measure exactly what patterns of exercise are the most effective. We will have precise quantitative measures of how much "good" epigenes are activated by which exercise regime. We will be able to answer question such as, do women profit differently from different exercises than men? What is the optimum amount of time per day, the optimum amount of exertion, the best machines? How much exercise per week? Is there a level below which there is no benefit? Is there a level above which there is no additional gain? How rapid is the epigenetic response? Minutes? Hours? Days? What about the effects of drugs on epigenetic response to exercise? These are all questions that now could be answered with great precision.

If you ask any coach or athlete or fitness instructor, they all have very strong opinions on these topics, but little science to back it up. And it's easy to see why. Any parameter that can be measured now is so indirect that one can anticipate a huge variation in response, probably so great as to be statistically meaningless. But directly measuring the responsible gene products means not having to rely on personal recall, or sloppy record keeping or any of the issues that make human subjects such difficult experimental material. You're probably wondering when we will have really solid data on epigenetic effects on exercise. This is simply an educated guess, but I think it will be quite soon, not 15 years in the future.

11

Aging: The End Game

Last scene of all,
That ends this strange eventful history,
Is second childishness and mere oblivion,
Sans teeth, sans eyes, sans taste, sans everything.
    —William Shakespeare, "The Seven Ages of Man"

The Story Concludes

As we've moved along in our epigenetic detective story, we've seen a raft of diseases that were traditionally thought to be the result of a combination of environmental and genetic forces, yet are now recognized to also find their origins in an epigenetics component. We have also seen that the risk of many of these conditions increases with age. Now we want to turn our consideration to the aging process itself, and ask if epigenetic factors may be contributors to the inevitable decline and final demise that is the inescapable consequence of the human condition.

Shakespeare gives us a brutally poetic portrayal of a process that we usually don't like to think about or talk about, but we certainly don't want to give him the last word on this topic. It turns out we know a lot more about aging than folks did in his time, and we know that epigenetic forces play an important role.[1] But how does epigenetics contribute to aging and what can we conclude about its nature? We come back to the same question; how do these forces play out against one another to produce the phenomenon? And if we understood the aging process, could we halt or even reverse it?

Ideas About Aging

As a non-scientific explanation, when people are asked, "what did your elderly relative die of?" the response often is, "He died of old age."

But this is not an explanation, this is a tautology that avoids an explanation. The person died because his body could no longer support life, and he succumbed to a heart attack, or infection, or diabetes, or cancer or a myriad of bodily failures that we associate with the aging process. So the question is, why did his body become progressively weaker over decades, and what were the fundamental forces that that finally ended his existence?

You might think that aging is a consequence of being a complex machine, and that all complex machines eventually wear out, the way cars and appliances and computers and airplanes do. But this is simplistic. For one thing, toasters don't self-repair. Our bodies have an astonishing capability of renewal and repair, and they are immensely more complex than any of our mechanical devices. We now know that all our body parts contain a special class of cells, known as stem cells, and that these keep cranking out replacement parts throughout the life of the individual. Even in the brain, nerve cells are replaced, an action that was previously believed not to occur.

But multicellular creatures seem to run the gamut in the longevity sweepstakes. We know that all mammals age, but there is a tremendous spread in maximum documented ages. For a human that number is 122; for mice, four years; for the forest shrew, two years; for dogs, 29; elephants, 86. But tortoises are known to live to 190, and whales may live 250 years.

These are snotty faced youngsters compared to giant sequoias, one alive and robust at 3,000 years. A Great Basin Bristlecone Pine, in the Sierra Nevada mountain range in California, has been recorded to be 4800 years old. Some multicellular organisms may be immortal, such as lobsters, which don't appear to decline in vigor, since they retain their ruddy manhood year after year, like an aquatic, claw-endowed Hugh Hefner.[2]

Bear in mind that these are maximum life spans, and average life spans for wild populations of plants and animals are much, much lower. Disease, accident and predation greatly limit their average lifespan. For humans, the 20th century saw a great increase in average lifespan in the U.S. and other industrialized countries, from around 45 years at the turn of the 20th century to around 78 at the turn of the 21st. But throughout human history there does not appear to be an increase in maximum longevity. The oldest authentically documented human being was Jeanne Calment,[3] a French woman who died recently at the age of 122. Prior to the 20th century it was difficult, but not impossible, to obtain accurate data, because social security and retirement systems had not been put into law. There is a documented case of an individual from 1798 living to 103, and another living to 110 from the year 1898 (all from Wikipedia).

With the rise of industrialization average longevity increased, mainly due to the establishment of public health measures (improvements in sanitation, clean water delivery, and better quality diet) rather than medical advances.[4] But this means that a large segment of the population now reaches the age at which they are susceptible to age related diseases, including Alzheimer's, cancer and cardiovascular disease.

The fact that for different mammalian species there is a clearly defined maximum lifespan has led many investigators over the years to conclude that aging was a programmed process, something built into the genes, a clock that would run out at a defined time. Many theories of aging were built on an evolutionary argument, based on the premise that if older members of the population were eliminated, this would leave space in the same ecological region for their offspring, so they wouldn't be crowded out by their parents. According to this theory, this would allow the production of newly invigorated members, generation after generation, constantly changing and adapting to new circumstances. Like all theories of aging this one has a lot of problems. One of the strongest objections to it is the fact that in the wild the vast majority of members of a species die long before they reach their maximum life span, due to predation, accidents, and disease, so it seems superfluous to have a genetic program to get rid of them. Another issue is the traditional belief that evolution works only at the level of the individual, meaning that after a member of a species completes their reproductive cycle, whether they lived or died would be irrelevant to increasing their contribution of genes to the next generation.

There are three major genres of aging theories, and many, many variations, up to 300,[5] so there's no shortage of people willing to go out on a limb on this topic. They can be roughly divided into three categories; (a) a genetic mutation concept, (b) a wear and tear category, and (c) the waste and junk accumulation group.

Wear and Tear

This is the "old Chevrolet" concept of aging—the theory that parts of cells, organs and the body in general wear out over time from constant use. It appeals to us, because we're all accustomed to seeing machines all around us wear out and reach a point where no amount of duct tape can hold them together. The theory was originated by August Weismann, a German scientist, back in the 19th century; the fact that we're even able to entertain theories from 130 years ago is either a tribute to Weismann's brilliance or a rather sad commentary on how slowly the field of aging research has progressed.[6] There is some experimental evidence for this idea, but it has not fared well over the years.[7] It is hard to reconcile this theory with the observation that mammalian life spans vary over such a wide range, and that some organisms don't seem to age at all. How could it be that whales are better than mice at maintaining their machinery in good repair? While it is clear that our bodies seem to experience a lot of wear and tear with the passage of the years, many commentators have opined that this is an effect rather than a cause of aging. Indeed, our bodies are actually very good at repairing broken bones or damaged tissues, and there is no logical reason why we should be cursed with the gradual loss of this capacity over time. In fact, salamanders are complex, highly differentiated creatures, and they are famous for their ability to regenerate entire amputated limbs![8] Most theorists agree that there no logical necessity for living organisms to wear out and not repair their damage, and as the examples listed above show, there are many multicellular organism that appear to be immortal, or close to it.

Accumulation of Junk

This is another group of theories that has not stood the test of time particularly well. The basic concept is that insoluble proteins accumulate in cells over the life of the individual, causing them to malfunction. When the level of accumulation passes a critical point, the organs have so many dead or underperforming cells in them that bodily systems begin to fail, and eventually the organism can no longer survive.

One of the main candidates for junk status is a pigment called lipo-fuscin, which is a cellular metabolic byproduct. Because it is insoluble, it accumulates with age.[9] It forms yellowish-brown pigment granules due to the oxidation of protein and lipid residues, and accumulates over the long term in various tissues within the lysosomes (small bags of enzymes that degrade unwanted molecules) of cells. It is known to build up in the muscles of elderly individuals, and could presumably cause the muscle cells to lose their appropriate function. It also accumulates in nerve cells and could compromise their performance. With advancing age, non-dividing, lipofuscin-loaded cells become increasingly unable to participate in the production of ATP, the energy molecule of the cell, leaving less and less capability for normal function, finally resulting in cell death. Lipofuscin is not the only nasty possibility that could gum up the works. Intracellular "garbage" of all types is not completely broken down and may accumulate over decades in long-lived species. Of course this theory, like many others, has a lot of holes in it. Once again we could turn the argument around and argue that the accumulation of lipofuscin and other junk is an effect rather than a cause of aging.

Somatic Mutation Theory of Aging

This is the idea that "mutations" accumulate in the DNA of body (or somatic) cells over the lifetime of the individual, gradually obliter-ating critical functions so that cells eventually fail. Here we're using the term "mutation" in a broad sense to include any kind of damage or alter-ation to the hereditary program, so these changes could be genomic or epigenomic.

When a significant amount of cellular loss occurs, vital organ sys-tems will no longer function, and at a critical point, survival is compro-mised.[10] Since these changes do not occur in the germinal cells (that give rise to the egg and sperm) they will not be passed on to subsequent generations. These changes in cells could explain the many diseases that age is akin to, including cancer, cardiovascular disease and neurological disorders. The fact that all these conditions are also associated with epi-genetic modifications strongly suggests a tight relationship between epigenomics and aging.

Dr. Denham Harman, now a professor emeritus at the University of Nebraska Medical Center, developed one of the early theory of somatic mutations in 1954. This is the "free radical theory of aging," that highly reactive compounds in the cell, known as free radicals, cause damage over time, driving the aging process. The study of the aging process appears to have had a salutary effect on Harman, now 98 years old. Harman is generally acknowledged as the "father of the free radical theory of aging."

A part of this theory is that a timer is built into it, in order to explain the fact that mammalian species have tightly defined maximum life spans. So this would suggest that these mutations accumulate more rapidly in short lived animals, such as mice, than in long lived animals, including humans and very large mammals. There is some evidence that the genomes of long lived animals are more stable than those of short-lived species. There are many investigations aimed at testing various predictions of the theory, and they have yielded mixed results.

Since this theory was first proposed, there has been a mountain of research aimed at supporting or refuting it. However, the vast majority of studies were done at a time when the epigenome was not recognized as a target for aging research. There are new studies that have included epigenetic changes in the aging analysis, and these are producing exciting results.

Although I call this the mutational theory of aging, it is probably more appropriate to think of it a general theory of damage to the hereditary apparatus, the concept that as an individual develops from a fertilized egg to an adult and then on to an inevitable decline, damage accumulates in the genetic program, which must now be thought to include epigenomic changes.

The Limited Lifespan of Human Cells in Culture

One observation that supports the concept of an "aging program" is the fact that when human cells, known as fibroblasts, are taken from the skin of a donor, and placed in plastic flasks with an appropriate nutrient medium, they have been shown to possess a limited lifespan.

135

The cells will undergo about 50 divisions, and then cease dividing. This experiment has been repeated thousands of times, in laboratories all over the world, and was first accomplished by Dr. Leonard Hayflick in 1965 at the Wistar Institute in Philadelphia. This phenomenon eventually became known as the "Hayflick Limit" and the observation has held up well over time. In a long series of experiments extending over a number of years, Hayflick and many other scientists demonstrated that there was an intrinsic program in the cells, and that altering the media or other growth conditions did not affect this Hayflick Limit. However, cells taken from older individuals were able to complete fewer and fewer generations, depending on the age of the donor, so the story was internally consistent, repeatable and made good sense, something we always like to see in a scientific model. In addition, cells from long-lived birds are able to complete more divisions in culture than cells taken from short-lived mammals, which also argues that the Hayflick Limit is a profound and basic property of multicellular animal species, and not some irrelevant observation of a pathological response of cells to their conditions of culture.[11]

Hayflick's work had a tremendous impact on the field of cell biology and aging research, as has been noted on many occasions.[12] His original papers, written with his colleague Paul Moorhead, have been cited thousands of times. The molecular basis is now much better understood (see next section). Interestingly, Hayflick over the years has been outspoken and very critical of "Methuselah" societies that want to do away with normal aging. He has been extremely critical of the feasibility and desirability of reversing the aging process, which provoked critical rebuttals.[13]

Telomeres

The very brief picture of the aging process that I have presented here has undergone a profound revamping in recent years resulting from the many advances that have been made in the molecular biology of aging. Perhaps the most essential discovery has been the telomere, now a part of the genetic material that has been thoroughly investigated and found to play a critical role in the cellular aging process. The concept was introduced back in the 1930s by Herman Muller, the discoverer of the mutagenic effects of X-rays that I introduced you to in Chapter 3 (see, I told you he was brilliant! See Chapter 3).[14] It comprises sequences of DNA located at the ends of the chromosomes, and it is absolutely essential for cell survival. Muller knew this, because he had produced many different strains of mutant flies by blasting them with X-rays and then studying their offspring. If he examined the chromosomes in many fruit flies that had been zapped with X-rays, he found that the genetic material of the progeny could endure all sorts of really brutal trashing, but one thing that they couldn't tolerate was the loss of the very ends of the chromosomes. So Muller recognized that the ends of chromosomes protected them from destruction and these ends were unique in some way. Of course, back then DNA hadn't been discovered and Muller had no way of knowing that he had made another Nobel Prize winning discovery. Similar observations were made in corn by Barbara McClintock, then at the University of Missouri at Columbia.

Much later it was determined that telomeres are repeating sequences of DNA, up to thousands and thousands of bases long, situated at the ends of the chromosomes. They don't code for any genetic messages, so they don't direct the synthesis of any protein, but rather behave as a buffering material, sort of like a protective bumper on a truck. Telomeres are maintained by a molecular complex known as telomerase which facilitates their copying, otherwise they replicate improperly and lose some of their sequences in every cell division, and eventually the chromosomes will be gnawed down and irreversibly damaged. This has been studied in normal skin cells taken from human patients, and it has been observed that over the course of many cell divisions the cells lose their telomeres and eventually their ability to divide. It is now recognized that telomeres play a central role in both tumor formation as well as the processes of cellular and organism aging.[15]

Because it is now possible to genetically engineer mice with specific genetic alterations, scientists have the opportunity to test hypotheses of gene function in way that they could only dream of a generation ago. For example, a mouse constructed to lack a critical molecule of the telomerase complex is unable to maintain telomere integrity and shows symptoms of premature aging. Such animals show organ decline and damage similar to that which takes place during the normal aging process.[16]

Epigenetics and Aging

I hope that this very brief orientation will give you a feeling for the concept of aging, and the research and theorizing that has taken place regarding this topic. It is fascinating and contentious, and we still have much to learn. But the central question is: "What is the connection between epigenetics and aging, and even if we don't have a complete understanding of the fundamental cause of human aging, can epigenetics add to this understanding, and most important, does epigenetics offer the possibility to halt or even reverse the aging process?"

I believe we can address this series of questions in the affirmative. As I have pointed out, there may be no single answer to the aging conundrum, and the basis of aging likely resides in a number of interacting causes. I suggest that an epigenetic basis may be a major component of this understanding. But in proposing a role for epigenetic participation, there is a fundamental point that must be noted.

We have seen throughout our story that DNA is noted for its stability; once mutations occur, they are fixed and not easily reversible. Epigenomic changes are much more frequent than mutations in the base pair reading of the DNA code, and they can be reversible, returning to their original configuration. Could this be a path to a reversal of the aging process?

In the first place, there's a lot of evidence demonstrating that as aging proceeds, damage accumulates in the DNA in the form of breaks, changes in the sequences of genes, rearrangements, loss of telomeres, and a general wearing down of the genetic program to a point where cell death becomes widespread. At the same time, changes in the chromatin, the protein associated with the DNA, are taking place, and these changes have epigenetic consequences. As stated earlier, we are looking at a shifting, morphing association between the DNA and the proteins; this association affects the architecture of the genetic apparatus. What's more, the stability of the DNA and the expression of the genes can be controlled through reversible chemical modifications of histone or modifications of DNA itself. Amongst the most prominent posttranslational modifications are histone acetylation and histone or DNA methylation.

This is what we mean when we refer to the dynamic state of the genome and epigenome, and this is why we cannot understand the control of the hereditary blueprints as they age without taking this genome/epigenome relationship into account. There is an ongoing process of age-related alterations occurring, but the epigenetic changes are reversible. This level of compaction and expression can be modified by specific enzymes, and the process is driven by the accumulation of errors in the DNA replication as the organism ages.

Will a Knowledge of the Epigenome Lead to a Conquest of the Aging Process?

Leonard Hayflick and his colleagues who have investigated aging over a number of decades have argued emphatically that it is impossible as a violation of physical laws to eliminate aging.[17] Hayflick states that aging is the result of random, accidental damage leading to a general loss of working molecules over time, and that the stability of these molecules is determined by the genes. So over time, more and more errors accumulate in the genome, more and more faulty molecules are produced, the ability of the organism to function declines until finally death occurs. Long-lived species would have evolved genes that program more robust, stable proteins, so it takes them longer to wear down. Since it takes large animals much longer to grow to maturity, give birth and raise their young, they would have to have better systems of maintenance and repair, so these would be the determinants of longevity. This process would be governed by the genome.

However, some recent epigenetic studies suggest that Hayflick's model may not be entirely accurate. A group in France[18] has been able to introduce what they call a "six gene cocktail" into cells that had almost exhausted their 50 generation of growth, or into cells from very old people (centenarians). You won't get this cocktail at your local pub, and the price will not go down during Happy Hour. The genes employed had been widely studied and are known to be important in the control of growth and healthy gene expression. To make the cocktail, they are put into the vectors that serve as the bearers of genetic information.

In both cases, the cells were at the end of their tether; they showed every indication of being tired and worn out. The appearance of the cells and the measurement of a number of physiological properties all were clear indications of their geriatric condition. But the treatment with the cocktail of genes reverses their senescence, and the cells now appear to be indistinguishable from human embryonic stem cells. These genes are introduced by patching and splicing the genes into the vehicle (referred to in the trade as a vector) for getting the genes efficiently into the cells. Once the genes enter into the cells they integrate into the cells' genomes and become a normal part of their genetic makeup. This is standard technology these days for studies in the basic medical and clinical sciences.[19]

This work suggests that it may be possible to use a patient's own cells to make embryonic stem cells that possess all the potential of cells taken from embryos. Yet these cells are completely compatible with the patient's own immune system, since they came directly from him. So in the future it may be possible to treat diseased organs or tissues, replacing them with renewed cells, grown from the patient's revitalized cells.

I corresponded with Hayflick on the claim of the French group that they were able to reverse the aging of human fibroblasts through their gene therapy intervention, since it seems to contradict his views on the aging process. His response was curt and to the point: "Any sensational claim as this research makes demands confirmation. Until that happens I remain a skeptic."

Hayflick's response motivated me to contact the French workers. Dr. Jean-Marc LeMaitre is the head of the team that published the studies on reversing aging through a gene therapy protocol. He stated that while Hayflick had established that normal human cells in culture undergo a loss of the ability to divide over time, the cells accumulate epigenetic changes during this period that affect their ability to express their normal gene profile. Since this profile can be reversed by their cocktail of growth factors, it means that accumulation of somatic mutations cannot explain cellular or tissue aging (15).

Gargling from the Fountain of Youth

There is no illness that is more subject to unabashed quackery than the aging process. Whether it is stem cells, human growth hormone, vitamin supplements, special diets, cosmetics, or exercise regimes, there is no road that has been left untraveled by the devious mind of man. Whole species of iconic mammals are now pushed to the brink of extinction to feed the superstitions of aging Asian millionaires.[20] While some may produce some transitory feeling of youthfulness, there is no authentic treatment for aging that exists now. And it is unlikely that there will be any that will benefit people old enough to read these words.

There are years of research ahead before we can routinely treat patients with stem cell therapy for aging disorders or any other disease. But at least we can say that the results are encouraging and there appears to be no fundamental barrier or law of nature that would prevent these therapies from being carried out. Finally it is important to recognize the role of epigenetics in the aging process and the escape from aging. When the promoters of these genes in the six gene cocktail that reverses the senescent cellular properties are demethylated, the genes are expressed and the cells can assume a "young" phenotype so we know that the gene weren't lost or damaged or degraded, they were simply epigenetically modified. Exactly how this process occurred and how it was regulated are complex questions that will have to be answered if we are to really control this process and employ it to build therapies for the future. It will take independent confirmation and years of effort to establish these findings on a firm footing.

12

Epigenetics to the
Ends of the Earth

The Perils of Environmental Research

I've touched on the linkage of epigenetics to environmental concerns throughout this book, but I want to give you some details about where the limits of our knowledge lie and how scientists attack this problem. The exposure of humans and animals to substances and stresses in the environment that could constitute an epigenetic risk is paramount as we try to understand the risks of epigenetic damage and build a meaningful response, as I'll consider in the final chapters.

Environmental questions are especially difficult to investigate. When we study the adverse effects of chemicals and other agents on plants, animals and humans, we are moving into an area that is rife with controversy. It may be extremely problematical to transpose findings made under controlled conditions in the laboratory to the field, and it is difficult to extrapolate from studies that show damage with high doses of epigenetic chemicals in the laboratory to observations in the environment where exposures may be much lower, difficult to document and may be intermittent and indeterminate.

Furthermore, cause and effect relationships gleaned from nature are often difficult, if not impossible, to establish. For instance, if we see that there is an increase in the incidence of autism among children born to farm workers exposed to suspected epimutagens, how can we be sure that the increase is not due to some other cause, such as infections, poor nutrition or the effects of poverty in general? Simply because two things occur together (for instance autism and pesticide spraying) this does not mean that one is the cause of the other. Clearly it takes a lot of good detective work to build on our hypothesis.[1]

Another problem is a political one. Most of the chemicals and other substances that are believed to cause epigenetic changes are there for a reason; they were developed for industrial or pharmaceutical or agricultural purposes, which means that there is a corporation somewhere whose feelings are going to be hurt if they are accused of producing and distributing a chemical that may cause serious diseases.[2] It is in their interest to fund research studies and to generate reports that argue for the safety of their products. Sometimes they're in the right. Their studies may be properly performed and rigorous and subject to scathing peer review. But as I pointed out in the last chapter, good science means repeating these studies, and approaching the question in a different fashion, to make sure you're not fooling yourself or other people.

One of the best scientists I know told me one time that whenever he does an experiment and gets the result that he is expecting, he immediately sits down and tries to figure out all the ways he could have got the "right" (desired, expected) answer for the wrong reason. I can't imagine that when a research team at a major corporation finds that their leading insecticide does not cause damage to the mammalian reproductive system, that they are going to sit around a conference table for hours on end designing experiments that will disprove the data that they all have been praying for.

Screening for Mutations: The Early Years

I want to engage you with some more antediluvian history concerning studies on mutational changes. Back in the 1960s scientists throughout the world were engaged in finding ways to test for the mutagenicity of radiation, chemical and other agents in our environment. There was a lot of interest in radiation at that point (remember this was the height of the Cold War) and the mouse was a widely used experimental tool. Oak Ridge National Laboratory and the Jackson Laboratory in Bar Harbor, Maine, received mountains of federal largesse and pursued huge programs to study the effect of various agents in literally millions of mice. People were also interested in compounds such as caffeine, and mammoth studies were performed to see if caffeine and other food additives caused mutations in the mouse. The studies established early on mammalian genome is quite stable; spontaneous mutations rates are quite low and caffeine did not appear to be a mutagen or a cancer causing agent.[3]

Despite gargantuan investigations with the massive research budgets available during the 60s, scientists found it impossible to test large numbers of substances for their mutagenicity in mice. Remember, we're talking about thousands and thousands of suspect chemicals, then and now. So a group at the UC Berkeley, headed by Dr. Bruce Ames, developed a test system in bacteria that they argued would save lots of time and money and allow many compounds to be evaluated.[4] It came to be known as the Ames Test, and it consisted of a number of features; a special strain of bacteria with a number of genetic mutations that made it perform accurately, rapidly and economically. It also involved the use of a soup of liver enzymes that could transform certain compounds into mutagenic substances, as would happen in an intact mammal.

So using this very nice system, the test bacteria were exposed to a range of concentrations of many different suspected chemicals, and mutations were recorded as colonies appearing on plates of nutrient agar. The media were designed in such a way that the bacteria could not survive unless specific mutations in these target genes had occurred in their genomic DNA.

The Ames test was widely used during this period, and Ames and his collaborators published many papers, looking at hundreds and hundreds of chemicals, both synthetic and naturally occurring, that were implicated in causing cancer or mutations. Over the course of many years they came to the conclusion that the prior, standard tests were uninformative, because the doses of the chemical they used were much higher than the amounts that plants, animals and humans encountered in the real world. Ames stated that there are thousands and thousands of naturally occurring substances that will produce a positive result if applied in high enough concentrations.[5] This would suggest that the natural repair mechanisms that cells possess to repair damaged DNA keep the potential mutagens at bay, preventing significant problems at the low concentrations in which they ordinarily would occur in the environment.

In support of this interpretation, the American Chemistry Council, a lobbying group for the industry, has argued that current exposure levels for BPA (a possible epimutagen, see below) are reasonable and there is no evidence for any effect on human populations. They have cited on their website a review of the literature concerning BPA by a large collaborative group of German scientists including toxicology experts, governmental health and safety specialists, pharma representatives and private consultants.[6] The judgment of the authors is: "Overall, the Committee concluded that the current tolerable daily intake for BPA is adequately justified and that the available evidence indicates that BPA exposure represents no noteworthy risk to the health of the human population, including newborns and babies." However, if the authors of the paper (published in 2011) thought that this would end the controversy over the health effects of BPA, they were sorely mistaken. In the intervening period (2011 to 2013) I find 179 peer-reviewed publications on the health effects of BPA on the Medline search engine. Some of these studies directly contradict the conclusion reached by the German group of investigators.[7]

According to Dr. Dana Dolinoy, of the University of Michigan, Ann Arbor, "This issue is far from settled. After the German report was published, an American group published a rebuttal, which prompted another rebuttal from the Germans and a re-rebuttal from the Americans. The people at the U.S. National Institute of Environmental Health Sciences have formed a consortium and produced some really helpful guidelines on conducting research on BPA."

Screening for Epimutagens

Ames and his collaborators developed mutation screening technology four decades ago. I have talked a lot in these pages about the history of genetics because the whole idea of the "paradigm shift" requires that we understand what was there before the new paradigm was introduced. The critical point is that genome mutation screening leaves unanswered the question of the existence of epimutagenic substances. The Ames test would not detect them, since although bacteria have epigenetic modifications, they use very different chemical reactions for methylation, and bacterial DNA doesn't use histones at all.

You will recall that I used the phrase "tsunami" to describe the chemical bath in which our society is awash, in the introduction to this volume. I did ask Ames his opinion and he referred me to a number of his publications. The conclusions drawn a number of years ago, that naturally occurring and synthetic mutagenic compounds do not constitute a significant health hazard, have been recently re-asserted.

Ames' views are shared today by a huge slice of the business community who never saw an environmental regulation with which they could live.[8] And for decades many scientists well qualified in the area of environmental mutagenesis would agree that our natural cellular repair systems are efficient enough, and the levels of DNA genomic mutagenic compounds in the environment are low enough that they do not constitute a significant risk.

Environmental Epimutagens

Even though the issue is a controversial one, there is a large body of evidence accumulating that the real risk is from the epimutagens, that they have not been appropriately classified, tested and monitored, and that even at the concentration present in the environment they may be contributing to the huge increases that we have seen in the catalogue of illnesses discussed in previous chapters.

Let's take a look.

We've looked at some environmental agents that may act as epimutagens elsewhere in this volume. Prominent among these are the heavy metals, including aluminum, arsenic, chromium, nickel, mercury and selenium. All of these heavy metal elements are well-known for their role in cancer causation and other diseases, and all are known to cause extensive epigenetic changes.[9]

Another class of compounds with significant epigenetic effects are the substances known as endocrine disruptors, which we've mentioned already.[10]

There are many, many chemical compounds that are classed as endocrine disruptors.[11] The list includes plastics components, insecticides, pesticides, steroid hormone analogues (similar but not identical molecules). As one of the most widely disseminated endocrine disruptors, BPA has been extensively studied for its possible role as an epimutagen. It could do this by binding to the cells, mimicking a hormone and botching up the signals that the hormone sends out through its epigenetic network. Or it could work directly through epigenetic mechanisms, affecting the epigenetic sites in genes that control hormone related functions. Shelby Flint and his colleagues at the University of Minnesota reviewed hundreds of studies evaluating the effects of BPA on wildlife, and they list many studies describing adverse effects of BPA on wild populations of birds, frogs, crustaceans and mollusks. I checked with Flint concerning his paper and he confirmed that his investigations do not distinguish a mechanism of BPA action. In either case, the fact that so many reports of adverse effects have appeared in the literature is certainly a reason for serious concern. Moreover, experts in the field suggest that the response to endocrine disrupting chemicals by invertebrates may be a warning of serious environmental disruption.[12]

It is important to bear in mind that response to hormones is a very ancient evolutionary signal. Hormone-like molecules run all through the entire kingdom of life. BPA and other chemicals widely dispersed throughout our environment could seriously affect growth and reproduction of thousands of species from the bottom to the top of the food chain with extremely widespread and unanticipated consequences.

Wildlife and Epigenetic Changes

We talked about the evidence that chemicals widely dispersed throughout the environment may cause epigenetic mutations, based on studies using tissue culture cells, lab animals and observations on humans. There is another approach, and that is investigations on wildlife. Although animal populations in a natural setting are very different from humans, they do provide more realistic circumstances, since we may have the opportunity to look at epigenetic changes brought on by very low concentrations of putative epimutagens, and we may be able to follow the path of these substances as they travel through the environment and the food chain.

Dr. Flint (referred to above) and his colleagues state that there are thousands of synthetic substances out there (sure sounds like a tsunami to me!) but their work focused on BPA because it is so widespread as a component of plastics, with 5.5 million metric tons produced in 2011.[13] There are now many studies on the effects of endocrine disruptors on both human populations and wildlife. Flint and his colleagues list about 50 studies in which BPA was shown to have profound effects on sexual development in many different aquatic wildlife, including many species of fish, insects, mollusks, sea urchins and crustaceans. Many other studies on domestic and wild birds, reptiles, mammals and amphibians show a range of malformations and sexual abnormalities.

Tales Too Troubling to Tell

Let me give you a flavor of some of the really bizarre accounts of environmental effects of endocrine disruptors on wildlife (believe me, there are lots more!). One involved starlings foraging on earthworms from garbage sites. The earthworms were heavily contaminated with estradiol (a female hormone, present in human wastewater), phthalates and BPA. When wild birds were fed this contaminated diet, the males had a significantly enhanced song repertoire; more complex, longer, a more appealing attractant for the females. Whereas you might think this is good for the birds, it is not. Bird song is an indication of overall robustness and males use it as a sort of oral Lamborghini to attract females. The better the song, the better overall genetic endowment of the potential mate. In fact, these males were less healthy than their untreated counterparts. So this is "false advertising"; the females will not pick the best mates, because their song and their other physical attributes don't match. So the next generation will be less fit than the previous. So this means that the best qualities of reproductive fitness will not be preserved in the species.[14]

Another really unusual environmental detective story involves endocrine disruptors driving masculinization in the female mosquito fish. When investigators studied fish living downstream from the discharge of a paper plant in Florida, they were observed to have male secondary sex characteristics.[15] The source was most surprising: a bacterial species that forms mats at the discharge site, converting a plant sterol in the paper waste to an extremely potent male hormone, androstenedione.

I point out these accounts because they are examples of some of the excellent detective work being done by systems biologists and ecologists, in which they work through complex chains of cause and effect, and because these patterns would never be uncovered without a lot of effort. Both the scientific literature and popular accounts are crammed with examples of the interdependency of plants and animal life within the biosphere, and the unexpected and disastrous results that can occur when the web of life is interrupted.[16]

Awash in Disruptors

These phenomena are not unique, and are being observed more and more frequently. Scientists have no idea of the total amount of steroid hormones from sources such as cattle feed lots and what gets flushed down your toilet,[17] nor is there any notion as to the overall amount of "hormone like" substances dumped into the environment from plastic and other industrial production and degradation. The total amount of environmental contamination with synthetic chemicals that give an estrogenic signal is not known, but it is vast by any measure. Data are sketchy and incomplete, but 45,000 metric tons of the weak estrogen, p-nonylphenol, were produced in 1976, and by 1982 the total annual production of all alkyl phenol polyethoxylates (compounds used in industrial processes) was estimated at 140,000 metric tons. They are toxic to many aquatic organisms. In 1993 BPA production in the United States was 640 million kg; of that, 44,000 kg (0.10 percent) was reported recycled, land filled, incinerated, or released in the environment. But this is just one compound. Plastic additives known as phthalates are generated at a level of 11 billion lbs/year; the antibiotic triclosan, used in soaps and toothpaste, one million lbs/year; pesticides, herbicides and fungicides 1.2 trillion lbs (with a "T") per year.[18]

Industrial cattle, hog and chicken production takes place on an unimaginable scale today, with accompanying massive pollution. One article lists 20 different studies in which environmentally contaminating endocrine disruptors cause a profound litany of reproductive damage, some so serious as to result in death, in animal species going all the way from pond scum (Daphnia) to humans.[19]

Drawing Conclusions

Endocrinologist Dr. Michael Skinner, who was quoted previously, asserts that one of the most dramatic causes for concern comes from the field of epidemiology in which environmental effects have brought about drastic changes in animal and plant populations over very short time frames. But these observations do not agree with a purely genetic determinism model, since many environmental agents don't directly affect DNA sequences. He adds that the abbreviated periods during which these changes took place are too short to agree with a model based on DNA-based mutations in the genome. This goes back to the argument that I made earlier that the DNA is quite stable, but the epigenome is notoriously fragile and unstable.

Skinner believes one of the major reasons for this disagreement concerning the cause of these changes is the fact that classic toxicology studies assume a linear relationship between dose of the chemical in question and the amount of damage. That is, if you give a big dose of a chemical to a test system you get a lot of damage, and if you apply less you get proportionally less damage. But now evidence is accumulating that at really low doses you may actually get more damage than conventional models predict, for reasons that are not clear. Since classic toxicological studies extrapolate from high doses to low ones, this can make interpretation of the result quite challenging.

Skinner is also troubled by the lack of reliable data on exposure of fetuses and newborns to putative epimutagens, given that rapid periods of development are envisioned to be the most fragile and sensitive to epigenetic damage. This may be another source for the conflicting results that have been reported over the years.

He expressed particular concern over the potential hazards of BPA. It is quite likely that epigenetic damage builds up over an extended period, perhaps the lifetime of the individual. This means that looking for epigenetic damage in a large population and then trying to correlate this amount of damage with serum or urine levels of BPA may not be meaningful. "BPA can cause changes in the highly sensitive mammary epithelium which 30 years later can translate into breast cancer. This is very difficult to track through classical toxicological studies. These are mechanisms that the traditional toxicologists are not going to like."[20]

Skinner argues that in terms of risk assessment it totally changes interpretation of all their tests, precipitating a lot of pushback from the establishment. Concerns over the possible hazards of BPA have been a strong driver of legislation, even though agreement on its risks is far from universal. Research by Skinner and others on animal models demonstrates that a mixture of plastic derived compounds, BPA and phthalates, can promote epigenetic inheritance of adult onset disease over several generations.[21] But Skinner doesn't see a path to easy solutions.

"Everybody wants to get rid of BPA but the replacement, known as BPS, has not been thoroughly evaluated. So we have to be careful and give the industry and science time to find an alternative. California has passed bans on BPA, but they are favoring a substitute compound that may be just as bad or worse."

Connect the Dots

It defies common sense to assert that our planet could be drowning in billions of pounds of substances that we know to be powerful epigenetic effectors, with no consequences to ourselves or to other living creatures. The evidence to the contrary is now overwhelming.

Connect the dots. Isn't that what they say? John Mclachlin of Tulane University connects them this way: "If male fruit bats are lactating in Malaysia, look for the environmental hormone. If there is a dramatic increase in the cases of premature breast development in Puerto Rico, look for the environmental hormone. And, if a 50-yr-old (male) mortician presents with (female sex characteristics) with no estrogen producing tumor, look for the environmental hormones."

13

Why Should You Care
About Epigenetics?

Many Things to Agonize About

Our civilization today is beset with problems, ranging from global, worldwide concerns to down and dirty, day to day, personal worries. With all these demons to keep us awake at night, what is it that sets epigenetics apart? Why should it represent a concern any more significant than the myriad other problems that beset our world?

If we were to add up "the sum of all fears" we'd find that each person has his or her own collection of individual disquiet. Much of these fears reflect the individual's private or political philosophy. Conservatives complain that religious values are eroding, that governments have moved into a tyrannical phase of dominance and that civilization is on a downward slide.

Climate change and environmental issues are of great concern for those of the liberal persuasion: Bill Mckibben is a leading environmentalist and spokesperson for the movement. In an article in *Rolling Stone* he wrote: "We have five times as much oil and coal and gas on the books as climate scientists think is safe to burn. We'd have to keep 80 percent of those reserves locked away underground to avoid that fate. This coal, gas and oil are still technically in the soil. But it's already economically above ground—it's figured into share prices, companies are borrowing money against it, nations are basing their budgets on the presumed returns from their patrimony. It explains why the big fossil-fuel companies have fought so hard to prevent the regulation of carbon dioxide—those reserves are their primary asset, the holding that gives their companies their value."[1]

For those of you who lack a strong set of political beliefs, meteor strikes are high on the list of things to agonize over. Although the chances of a dinosaur-decimating event (a really big asteroid striking the earth) are small, NASA scientists estimate that a meteor strike of 150 feet in diameter occurs on the average every thousand years. Such an encounter in a major city would definitely get people's attention.[2] Since our civilization currently lacks the technology to deter any meteor, large or small, NASA scientists recommend prayer in the event of a major incoming denizen from outer space.

There are plenty of other issues to keep you up at night. Species extinction is rampant and could result in the loss of 25 percent of the world's species of plants and animals by the end of the century. According to the World Wildlife Fund, "The rapid loss of species we are seeing today is estimated by experts to be between 1,000 and 10,000 times higher than the natural extinction rate."[3]

In our country we should include a gridlocked government, a devastating drought in the central U.S. that has been going on for at least a decade, a dysfunctional prison system, and an immigration crisis that sees little hope of ending. U.S. infrastructure is so badly deteriorated that critics rate it as a "D" grade, and claim that it will cost trillions to bring it up to the level of the European Union.[4]

Internationally, problems abound. Rampant, life threatening pollution of the air and water in China and India (which spreads far beyond the borders of these countries), overexploitation of the oceans[5] and other natural resources, mismanaged economies, the constant threat of nuclear war, chronic and ongoing unrest in the middle East.

We cannot leave this melancholy list without a mention of the U.S. health care system, since it forms such an integral part of our consideration of epigenetics and its health consequences. When any public discussion of U.S. health care takes place, the speaker prefaces his remarks by saying that ours is the best in the world. Whereas John Boehner, speaker of the House of Representatives and Mitch McConnell, Senate minority leader, have both made this statement on numerous occasions,[6] on the whole the U.S. does not rank well among industrialized countries. According to the World Health Organization's international ranking, the United States comes in as the 37th best health care system out of 191 countries. Another study by the Commonwealth Fund that included a smaller number of nations found the U.S.'s performance to be mediocre at best. "Compared with six other nations—Australia, Canada, Germany, the Netherlands, New Zealand, and the United Kingdom—the U.S. health care system ranks last or next-to-last on five dimensions of a high performance health system: quality, access, efficiency, equity, and healthy lives." See Figure 13.

International ranking of health care systems is an inexact science, but there is one datum that is inarguable and highly relevant to this discussion: the U.S. Healthcare system is far and away the most expensive in the world. While one can quibble over whether we are getting our money's worth, the high cost of U.S. medical care is an inescapable reality.[7]

Throughout these chapters we have seen over and over again that a variety of illnesses have increased in frequency over the years, especially in recent decades. We have also seen that all of these conditions

US spends two-and-a-half times the OECD average

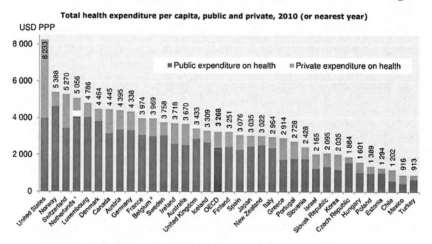

Total health expenditure per capita, public and private, 2010 (or nearest year)

1. In the Netherlands, it is not possible to clearly distinguish the public and private share related to investments.
2. Total expenditure excluding investments.
Information on data for Israel: http://dx.doi.org/10.1787/888932315602.

Source: OECD Health Data 2012.

Figure 13. Total per capita healthcare costs per country. Data demonstrate that the United States spends twice as much as the average for industrialized for healthcare; note correspondence). OECD (2012), *Health at a Glance: Europe 2012*, OECD Publishing. doi: 10.1787/9789264183896-en. Reprinted with permission (copyrights paid for).

are linked to epigenetic mechanisms, some, such as various cancers, inextricably so. Assuming that the conditions that are driving the increase in epigenetically related illnesses will continue to grow, this means that overall healthcare costs, already astronomical, will continue to rise. Looking into the future, it is clear that unless we understand fully and exert control over the epigenetic contribution to disease, the situation could become unmanageable in the near future.

Epigenetics: A Unique Challenge

I hope that in these chapters I have been able to convey a radical new picture of what is happening today in the life sciences, as new findings in the study of inheritance open up a pathway to our understanding of the structure of genes and epigenes and how they determine our phenotype. In conversations I have had with friends and colleagues, I have found that most people are fascinated by the concept, for its intrinsic novelty and interest.

Why should people who have never set foot in a laboratory, who are not scientists, and may even harbor a certain hostility toward science be enamored of epigenetics? There are a number of explanations for this, but the obvious feature of epigenetics is that it is intriguing in its own right. The fact that our hereditary makeup is much less fixed and stable than was commonly believed, the notion that epigenetic models can answer long-standing questions about what we inherit from our ancestors and what is programmed in by our environment, the suggestion that inherited conditions responsible for disease processes might be reversible, all of these are reasons explaining why an inquisitive mind would be swept away by this field and all it portends.

And there are other, more urgent reasons for why you should care about epigenetics; immediate, practical considerations dealing with disease and the survival of humanity. For if the epigenome is as fragile and evanescent as the evidence indicates, doesn't this mean that very slight changes in our environment could bring about alterations in the epigenome with profound and unwanted effects?

I point to a parade of concerns to anticipate a nagging question that the reader will raise: With so many issues (and so many that seem insurmountable) facing our society, why should epigenetics get any more consideration than the inventory of woes that I have laid out?

I argue that the threat of an overwhelming epigenetic health burden demands our attention in a special and unique way. There are many facts that I have marshaled to buttress this argument, and in these concluding chapters I will attempt to tie them together. Furthermore, as I will discuss later on, the threats of epigenetic damage to our health and to our environment are problems that we can actually do something about, rather than many of the other issues that I have mentioned that are so large and intractable that they appear to be insurmountable.

When the evidence concerning epigenetic hazards is laid out to the public, I believe that there will be an overwhelming push for action. This could take many forms; in the final chapter I will discuss these options. Today when a controversial issue comes to the attention of the public, it is hotly debated. After this, the issue moves to state and federal governmental bodies where it given due consideration. At this point the usual outcome is that no substantive action is taken to address the problem. This recalls the old adage: "When all is said and done, there is a lot more said than done."

The challenges of epigenetics are in no way as controversial as the many other current hot button issues that get buried by the rancor of our political system. This means that it could actually be possible to move ahead and make progress (what this "progress" is, I will define later). The discoveries in the field of epigenetics touch on many other areas of concern and form a major component of the puzzle of what the future holds for all of us. All of these challenges could overwhelm our ability to deal with them, but I believe that they can be understood, and finally brought under control.

Let's take a look at some these, and pull together information that we've laid out in previous chapters.

A Philosophical Commitment Drives Interest

Perhaps first on the list is the fact that epigenetics is in every sense a revolutionary reassessment of our place in nature, and as such it will change the way we think about the world and about ourselves. A few examples:

A Reconsideration of Lamarkianism

In the early chapters of this book I discussed the ideas put forth by Lamark in the early 19th century concerning the inheritance of acquired characteristics that were eventually rejected. Epigenetic inheritance excites our imagination because it suggests that in some cases, there could be a directive force: that is, certain environmental influences could cause epigenetic changes that could be passed to subsequent generations. Whereas epigenetic changes appear to offer the possibility that an organism could respond to environmental challenges by modifying genes through methylation, chromatin modification, or other epigenetic mechanisms and pass an adaptive change on to its offspring, this idea remains speculative. But behavioral studies on animals and humans strongly suggest that some epigenetic changes can be passed to the offspring, influencing the phenotype of the descendants. Most scientists feel that the epigenetic possibilities open a range of options for evolution, but do not modify the fundamental concept of Darwinian evolution.[8]

A Fragile Genetic Patrimony

I told you early on in this book that the genome tends to be quite stable. Although DNA-based (genomic) genes can mutate, this is a rare occurrence, and the long accepted consensus among the cognoscenti has been that these rare mutations are what drive evolution. But epigenetics suggests there is another side to the picture, that there is a fragile epigenetic component, and that it is subject to change without notice. It also suggests that the epigenome may play an important part in the origins of many disease states and that chemicals introduced into our environment may be responsible for adverse health effects by altering epigenomic sites.

Epigenetics and IQ

When we think of how genes and epigenes may control our characteristics, it is obvious that complicated human attributes, such as intelligence, could not be controlled by a single gene, but rather there must be a very complex system consisting of many genes, interacting together.[9] And to the genomic contributions we must add the environmental and epigenetic inputs, resulting in the three way interactive pattern. Studies on large populations in which "high IQ" and "low IQ" groups were compared have demonstrated that there are slight differences in DNA sequences in many genes, perhaps thousands. No gene variants have been found that individually made large contributions to IQ differences[10] (see Figure 14). These experiments are performed by large scale sequencing of DNA and looking for consistent differences between the two groups.

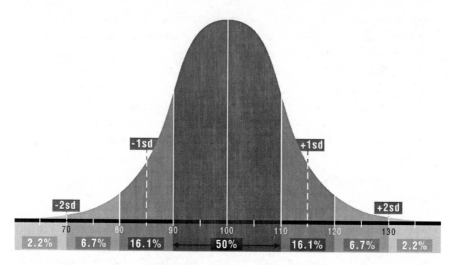

A Standard Bell Shaped Curve

Figure 14. Bell shaped curve. The bell-shaped curve, or normal distribution, is a classic description of how values are distributed about a mean. In this context IQ is influenced by many factors, and the average value will be the most frequent value. Normal distributions are the foundation of statistics and are extremely important in every branch of science. Drawn by Garima Naredi for this book.

I previously pointed out that twin studies suggest that IQ variation in human populations is determined anywhere between 30 percent and 70 percent by genetic input, and that the remainder is due to environmental contributions. These studies have yielded such disparate results that they are not terribly informative, and all we can conclude is that both heredity and environment play a role in determining our intellectual capabilities. But this is just common sense and constitutes a trivial observation. Who would argue against the proposition that heredity and environment make us who we are?

Recent (2012) studies point out a role for epigenetic modification of gene expression. Identical twins were compared for the amount of methylation in their DNA. It was found that a number of genes that are suspected of playing a role in IQ determination were differentially methylated in the two groups.[11] Stated another way, the results showed that for a given pair of identical twins, who differed substantially in their IQ scores, individual genes showed differing patterns of methylation. These results will have to be confirmed and expanded upon, but if they hold up, they would support the idea that the epigenome, the genome and the environment interact in a complex fashion to produce the overall intellectual phenotype of the individual.

This is completely different from the traditional picture of genes and environment, with its neat boxes for the two components. This new portrait is complex and messy, and suggests a melding and a running together of the three factors, playing back and forth throughout the life of the individual, and from generation to generation. This could mean that an individual's genotype will mold and create his environment, in the fashion that a individual with a robust, athletic phenotype would be drawn to an environment that nurture these abilities, and in turn, athletic prowess could feedback into the epigenome, influencing expression of specific alleles.

And you can perhaps envision how two individuals with the same or nearly the same genetic endowment, could, in different environments, be pulled epigenetically in different directions. This model is supported by a good deal of evidence that we have seen in the course of these chapters. And it does lend support to the idea that the individual perhaps has more power over his existence than traditional ideas of nature and nurture would suggest. This view is shared by researchers in the field of cognitive psychology.[12]

There is now a substantial body of research demonstrating the role of epigenetic changes in response to exercise. As pointed out (Chapter 10), genes are activated in direct response to exercise to produce the proteins that build fitness. These observations argue that the individual responds to his environment on a molecular level, and suggests that we have control over our fates in a manner that is much more direct and powerful than the conventional notions that assumed that hard work would lead to success in athletics, artistic performance, intellectual attainment or in the pursuit of so many goals that drive our lives.

A PERSONAL CONNECTION

Most people who have a driving personal interest in a disease are motivated by a connection through a close friend or relative who suffered from that disease. There is a huge presence in this country of private foundations, started by individuals motivated by desperation, inspiration, frustration or altruism who sought to establish an organization to prevent others from enduring what they have been through.[13] There are foundations for AIDS, cancer, Parkinson's disease, Alzheimer's disease, diabetes, muscular dystrophy, multiple sclerosis; virtually all of the diseases catalogued in these pages. I don't know of a single inherited disease that has been described in the scientific literature for which there is not a foundation dedicated to its basic research and treatment.

But the federal government is the main supporter of health research. The federally funded National Cancer Institute's budget request for 2012 was $5.2 billion, whereas the American Cancer Society, the largest U.S. non-governmental non-profit focusing on cancer, raised around $900 million in the period 2009–2011. The Susan G. Komen Foundation spent $66 million on research and research-related activities in 2011. Not chump change by any stretch, but this comparison illustrates how much more powerful the IRS is than a fun run when it comes to raising money to drive megaprojects.

Despite the small size of their resources when compared to the feds, private foundations that target various diseases perform a very important function. Because they are small and nimble, they have much greater freedom to dispense seed funds for imaginative projects that are exciting but may have a high probability of failure. The NCI and other federal governmental funding agencies tend to focus more and more on large scale efforts and research centers with huge budgets. This is because they perceive many of the questions facing science today to be resolvable only through massive endeavors, for which the human genome project serves as a model. The effort to map the human brain has been highly touted by President Obama, and it will be his highest priority item in health sciences research policy as he struggles to move NIH forward during the remainder of his term.

However, it may not be the best mechanism for expanding our knowledge as to how the brain works. As we have discussed, there is a growing body of knowledge connecting mental disorders and normal mental functioning with epigenetic mechanisms. This work is still in its early stages, but we are only beginning to understand the role of epigenetic controls in the functioning of the brain. At this time it is not clear that a vast and costly brain mapping project is the best way to understand the nature of thought, memory, personality and human individuality. This approach may be similar to trying to send a manned mission to Mars without a solid knowledge of Newton and Einstein's laws of motion and physics.

Don't take my word for it. According to the *New York Times,* a group of the world's leading neuroscientists have proposed a number of alternative approaches that they argue are more informative and could bring a better understanding of the brain at a lower cost.[14]

The small foundations can be looked upon as the venture capitalists of the non-profit sector. The private foundations, by funding dicey ideas, can give the "mom and pop" laboratories the opportunity to produce the data that will convince the big dogs that an idea is worth pursuing. Furthermore, because they are constantly soliciting funds, their activities constantly raise public awareness of diseases in a manner that governmental agencies cannot do. It would be most unusual to see a fun run sponsored by NIH, or a cocktail party for wealthy movers and shakers with the proceeds going to the National Science Foundation. Yet these approaches are ideal for small foundations anxious to generate public awareness and raise consciousness at the same time.

After my ringing endorsement of the power of private foundations, you may wonder if there are any that focus on epigenetic associated diseases. It turns out there are. For example, the Michael J. Fox Foundation for Parkinson's Research is funding a project aimed at drawing a link between environmental factors driving epigenetic changes to genes implicated in Parkinson's disease. The website states: "The expected outcome of these studies is that we might identify differences in the epigenetic fingerprint in PD patients versus controls. Since epigenetic changes are a novel concept for a risk and disease modifying mechanism in

Parkinson's Disease that has not been tested to date, positive as well as negative results would greatly advance our understanding and foster future research efforts."[15]

Admonitions for driving epigenetics research through private foundations abound. "I propose that researchers in the epigenetics and sarcoma communities meet in the near term in order to define a strategic path for sarcoma-related epigenetics research," says Dr. Bruce Shiver, writing on the Liddy Shiver Sarcoma Initiative website.

The American Institute for Cancer Research funds epigenetic research "that explores the effects of food, nutrition, physical activity and body weight on the development, treatment and survival of cancer." For instance, one investigation funded by the foundation is "Epigenetics of genistein and/or soy isoflavone in breast cancer prevention."

Fragile X syndrome has an important epigenetic component, and The Fraxa Foundation supports research on this disease. Fragile X is the most common inherited cause of mental impairment and the most common known cause of autism. The condition is the result of a repeat expansion of a segment on the X chromosome (which appears in two copies in females and one in males). Neurological manifestations vary widely and include developmental delays, cognitive disabilities, and seizures.[16]

The Simons Foundation Autism Research Initiative, whose logo states: "Advancing Research in Basic Science and Mathematics," has indicated their willingness to support a variety of basic research investigations.[17] These include enquiries into the epigenetic basis of autism.

The University of Southern California Keck School of Medicine has funds available from the Whittier Foundation to support non-cancer team-led translational research projects, including epigenetic-based investigations. Joan's Legacy, a foundation dedicated to lung cancer research, especially varieties not associated with cigarette smoking,[18] supports a number of projects with epigenetic implications. The Thomas G. Labrecque Foundation is especially committed to early detection of lung cancer, including evaluation of methylation patterns as a possible early marker. The Kazan Foundation has funded research on the ZLC1 gene, a tumor suppressor gene that is epigenetically regulated in cases of mesothelioma, one of the most deadly cancers, closely associated with exposure to asbestos and cigarette smoking.

What Drives Epimutational Change?

This is the probably the most critical issue, the essential question raised by this book. I have argued that there is now solid evidence that changes in the epigenome introduced by industrial, chemical and pharmacological processes ("epimutagens") are contributing to damage reflected in large increases in a host of diseases in humans, and to a range of negative effects in animal populations. If this emerging body of evidence continues to build and expand, then at a certain point the case becomes overwhelming and our society must take action, to avoid grave consequences.

It is important to recognize that all the conditions and diseases covered in this book are the sum of multiple factors. I discussed this issue with Dr. Heather Patisaul, a member of the Biology Department at North Carolina State University. Her area of research is the steroid-dependent mechanisms which are responsible for the sexually dimorphic behaviors and brain circuits in mammals, including humans. She and her associates have done extensive research on the endocrine disruptors and their effects on development.

"It's very important to recognize that changes we are seeing in humans and in animal populations related to endocrine disruptors are the result of multiple factors," she stated. "One of the most disturbing of these trends is the early onset of puberty, which is occurring in many countries throughout the world. My position is that if it were simply a single agent, such as bisphenol A that we had to contend with, the individual might be able to deal with it, but when you add stress and other factors on top of it, you set up the population for adverse effects from these factors acting synergistically."

Patisaul asserts that you are not going to be able to find a unitary cause for the disturbing changes that we are seeing in animal and human populations. Endocrine disruptors are entering the environment from multiple sources, they act on different systems in different ways and their elimination will require their identification and assessment of the role that they play in different pathologies.

There are some diseases with an epigenetic component that are becoming less frequent, such as various cancers. There are others, such as Alzheimer's disease, in which factors unrelated to epigenetics (such as the increasing age of the population) may be part of the increase in the incidence of this condition. Nonetheless, careful epidemiological studies can allow us to separate out these contributions and determine the role of epigenetic changes.

Many Challenges, Not Much Time

In previous chapters I have presented a growing body of evidence supporting an epigenetic component for a wide range of disease conditions. As asserted earlier, this does not mean that these diseases are solely due to alterations in the epigenome. What it means is that epigenomic changes play a role, and in some cases a deciding role, in the onset of many diseases. It means that the genome, the epigenome and the environment are all playing back and forth on one another to generate an outcome. In some cases this may be a modulation of a normal process, in other cases it may portend the onset of a cataclysmic illness. While this playbook is still incomplete, it is well established and supported by a powerful body of research. This work consists of thousands and thousands of scientific papers in the best peer-reviewed journals. It is clear that it is no longer possible to discuss health and disease states in humans or in animals without taking the epigenome into account. It is no longer possible to argue the effects of pollution and the risks to the environment without recognizing the role of epigenetics in the web of our planet's totality of life.

Perhaps the most critical question today is to what extent the environment drives these inputs to the epigenome. In this case, environment refers to the exposure to drugs and other chemical substances, but is also may include availability of nutrients and even psychological and behavioral inputs. We have seen that based on studies on experimental animals and observations from famines in human populations, severe caloric restriction can bring on epigenomic changes that may be manifested decades after in utero exposure. And, as previously discussed, there is evidence accumulating that behavioral inputs, such as exercise, may cause epigenetic responses.[19]

I believe that the situation regarding epigenetic risk and the public hazard is comparable to debate over cigarette smoking. Cigarettes were known for years before the Surgeon General's report in 1964 to constitute a health hazard, yet for years before and after the report their health effects were debated. At a certain point the evidence became so overwhelming that even the cigarette manufacturers could not argue against it, and were reduced to specious arguments concerning the freedom of smokers to do what they wanted.[20] In a similar vein, at a certain point, the evidence supporting the damaging effects of epimutagenic agents will become overwhelming, and will force action.

Sorting out these cause and effect relationships will be a critical task for the coming years. As our understanding and knowledge of epigenetics grows, the regulatory decisions and the search for alternatives will become ever more critical, since so many of the chemicals released into the environment are important in the pharma, agricultural and industrial sectors. We will need the best and most extensive science to guide a new generation of environmental laws that take into account these discoveries. This will take a lot of time and money and commitment on the part of the government. But given the current gridlock of our political system, nothing will happen without the strongest pressure exerted on our political establishment by the public.

So in the final two chapters, I'm going to see if we can pull these ideas together and come up with a plan.

14

Pulling It All Together

The story that I have related here covers a lot of ground, putting together a picture of how modern medical science operates today and how so much of its efforts are focused on epigenetics. I talked about how information is gathered in life science research, the tools that scientists use, the personalities of many of the people at the forefront of discovery. I've talked about potholes on the road to innovation and what can go wrong. Now I would like to pull these concepts together and talk about the future of epigenetics, both from the standpoint of the science and from the viewpoint of the political, social, economic and cultural implications involved.

What We Thought We Knew

The scientific community is beginning to recognize that the forces that control our hereditary makeup are much more complex and nuanced than was believed only a few years ago. At the outset I laid out the conventional wisdom of the genome as a long linear tape of DNA that spells out messages. These messages are solid, sitting in the cell nucleus in isolated splendor. Complementary RNA copies are split off, and these move out from the nucleus into the cell cytoplasm and get together with some fancy machinery made out of RNA and protein to make protein molecules, the sum total of which makes us what we are. Admittedly, some genes are turned on and off in the life history of the individual, but this is pretty much a staid, comfortable kind of grandfatherly genome, not changing much, a predictable, easy to comprehend kind of genome, a genome that doesn't make waves. It was clear that many genes were activated and deactivated, as a fertilized egg transformed itself through a series of conversions into a fully formed indi-

166

vidual, but this was envisioned to work through controller genes that behaved as master switches, turning the protein coding genes on and off at the appropriate times.

This genome can change through mutations that affect the messages; these mutations are quite rare. The DNA molecules are knocked about and the words are slightly altered. When these rare mutations occur they can cause dreadful diseases (or have no effect at all), like sickle cell anemia and cystic fibrosis and Tay-Sachs disease. These diseases are brutal, and very difficult to treat, but they're rare. It's been known for a century that radiation and certain chemicals could increase the frequency of mutations and could cause cancers, and that these mutations in the genomes of different body cells could make them into rampaging tumors. But these were exceptional events; mutation in the egg and sperm were so rare that they were hard to measure, and although producing mutations in mice and fruit flies was well understood, it seemed like the marvelous built-in repair systems that our cells carried would protect us from all but the most egregious assault, such as that occurring during a nuclear war, or a cataclysmic industrial accident.

And a wealth of data supported this assessment. Exposure of the general population to industrial chemicals was at levels far below those known to cause mutations in experimental animals. Numerous assessments indicated that while farm workers, oil refinery workers and other groups may have suffered health effects from acute exposure to very high levels of these substances, there was no evidence that the overall health of the vast majority of Americans was affected by the wealth of chemical molecules that have been so important in their lives for generations. These conclusions were supported by testing of thousands of chemicals, both naturally occurring in plants, and synthetically generated. These studies showed that while many of these chemical could cause mutations in test systems, the dose required was higher, sometimes by hundreds of times, that which was present in the environment.

Cancer was another chapter in this appraisal. It was inescapable that massive doses of powerful carcinogens, delivered over a 30-year period could make the last years of a smoker's life into a living hell. But most other cancers were blamed on secular trends, either an act of God, or bad diet. The fact that cancer rates varied widely in countries throughout the world was thought to be due to dietary factors, since when people emigrated from one country to another and assumed the eating habits of their adopted land, their cancer rates came to reflect those of the natives. The accepted party line was that while a healthy lifestyle might lower somewhat the risk of cancer, there wasn't a lot that an individual could do beyond this to avoid cancer.

So cancer research focused on discovering more and more powerful drugs to treat malignancies once they were clinically detected. And this approach would make sense, if most cancers were the result of factors that couldn't be controlled, or only controlled with the greatest disruption of the individual's existence.

Likewise, in the case of a whole host of diseases, ranging from diabetes to mental disorders to cardiovascular disease, the origins were said to be complex. All these diseases appeared to have a strong genetic predisposition, based on twin studies. Yet the fact that identical twins were not 100 percent concordant meant that some differences in the environment, such as diet or other agents, were also responsible. For many disorders, the search for causes took on the aura of a religion. Autism has been blamed on many factors, in particular vaccination. Other diseases, such as bipolar disorder and schizophrenia have been blamed on bad parenting, even though no solid, consistent evidence could be mustered to support such claims.

What We Know

But what I have presented here is a radically new view of inheritance from the work of the epigenetics research community:

(I) The phenotype of virtually all living creatures consists of the genome comprising the DNA-based messages, the epigenome, a network of chemical compounds surrounding the DNA that modify the genome without altering the DNA sequences.[1] These chemical signals act as switches, turning on and off specific genes. They respond to external signals, emanating from the environment surrounding the organism. These three entities interact together in a complex pattern of cross talk, so that epigenomic signals are activated by environmental signals, and they in turn trigger the appropriate gene response. Under normal conditions complex organisms respond to these signals and a lively conversation ensues, resulting in the realization of a complex pattern of expression.

(II) There are three major epigenetic signaling mechanisms: DNA methylation, histone modification and microRNAs. The sequence: cytosine-guanine in the DNA may undergo a chemical reaction known as methylation, acting as an on/off switch for the genes. In addition there are repeating sequences of cytosine-guanine in the genome, known as CpG islands, which occur next to approximately 70 percent of human genes. The CpG islands are ordinarily not methylated but may be in abnormal situations.

(III) The conventional graphic depiction of the genome as a long straight line of information (like a long line of text in a written document) is not correct. Genes loop out in complex, three dimensional structures, bringing far-separated parts of the genome into close proximity with one another. The histone proteins associate with gene sequences to shut them off and modulate their expression. Their behavior is determined by methylation of the protein resulting in direct interactions between the histones and DNA. The mammalian genome cannot function without this three-dimensional structure.

(IV) Many disease states and conditions involving physiological responses that we do not consider to be diseases, such as aging, have been conclusively shown to have an epigenetic component. The evidence in support of this proposition is based on epigenetic regulation of genes that are involved in the expression of these altered states. The strongest body of evidence concerns the epigenetic contribution to a wide range of cancers. This does not mean that epigenetic factors are the lone component, but rather epigenetic input plays an important role in their expression. It is no longer possible to formulate an understanding of most diseases without taking epigenetics into the design.

(V) Diseases believed to have an epigenetic basis, including certain cancers, diabetes, autism, schizophrenia, bipolar disorder and Alzheimer's disease have increased in frequency dramatically in recent decades. These observed increases remain even when changes in diagnostic criteria and other factors are taken into account.

(VI) Since the end of World War II a vast number of chemicals have been introduced into the environment. In most cases little is known concerning their health effects. Many are known to be epigenetically active.

(VII) There is a large body of evidence that many abnormalities in experimental animals and wild populations of insects, fish, mollusks, crustaceans, birds and mammals can be induced by levels of chemical compounds at concentrations observed in the environment. Many of these agents are known to cause damage through epigenetic modifications.

(VIII) In humans a number of toxic agents that cause epigenetic changes have been linked to increases in cancer and numerous other diseases. Most of these studies have focused on DNA methylation and histone modification.

(IX) Most epigenetic modifications are wiped clean in each generation, so the egg and sperm that will be the new generation are free from the epigenetic changes that occurred to the individual during his lifetime. But there are examples of cases in which epigenetic change are passed to the next generation. This remains a contentious area.

(X) It is impossible to understand modern biology without a knowledge of epigenetics and its role in heredity.

What We Don't Know

Despite a mass of research findings, there is much work that needs to be done if we are to build a series of cause and effect relationships linking epigenetic modifications in specific genes and the expression of specific diseases. This means epigenetic modifications of gene expression need to be tied to particular diseases, and a solid mechanism needs to be established. This has proven vexing, since for most diseases, their basis is complex. But this doesn't mean that building this understanding is impossible, it is simply difficult. Solving these questions will require a true commitment and billions and billions of dollars in federal funding.

Perhaps the greatest and most frightening unknown is what is causing the increase in diseases with an epigenetic connection. There is much circumstantial and inferential data, but as yet there is no consensus that (for example) the increase in the incidence of autism is due to an increasing exposure to epimutagenic chemicals. The same holds true for the other conditions that I have argued have an epigenetic component. This question will have to be attacked from all angles; animal models, cell culture and human epidemiological studies.

It is not known what the difference is between the majority of genes and the genes that are epigenetically modified in a fashion that may be passed to the next generation. Because a cardinal rule of epigenetics has been that the slate is wiped clean in every generation, we should not expect epigenetic changes to be fixed. This should not occur and yet it does. This is a vital clue to our understanding of the epigenome and how it operates.

With a more detailed understanding of how epigenetic changes link to a particular disease, it should then be possible to develop epigenetic-based drugs that can treat these conditions. There are several drugs that interfere with methylation that are being used to treat cancers, but progress has been slow, and there are no FDA-approved drugs for treating other conditions.

One of the most significant challenges will be the need to develop drugs that are highly specific for targeted genes, yet do not interact with the rest of the epigenome.

Politics and Science

It is not the purpose of this account to lay out a step by step plan for resolving all the unanswered questions in the field of epigenetics (that would require a much longer book), but rather to indicate, in a general way, that we have much to do. The United States, the leader in science for the last 60 years, must be the leading country in this enterprise. Today there are signs that this may not happen.

We see a disturbing trend in the commitment of the American people and their leadership to the pursuit of science. For years, going back to the early days following the end of World War II, there has been an agreement between the political parties and the American people that science is an intrinsic good, and that the United States needs to lead the world in scientific discovery. During the 1950s up until the 1980s a combination of unwavering public support and superb congressional leadership allowed an unprecedented series of scientific accomplishments. But in the mid 80s this partnership weakened and eventually stumbled. Government funding for science has been flat since 2004 (with the exception of a onetime shot from the stimulus in 2009) and is now experiencing a precipitous collapse, dropping 18 percent from 2004 to 2013 (see Figure 15).

At the time of this writing, no 2014 budget has been passed, but the outlook is hardly encouraging. The senate request of $30.3 billion would represent a one percent increase above FY 2012 levels, but factoring in an inflation rate of 4.0 percent between FY 2012 and FY 2014, the figure is a 2.9 percent decline in R&D funding from pre-sequester spending. The house budget, on the other hand, calls for a 30 percent cut, to *ca.* $20 billion.

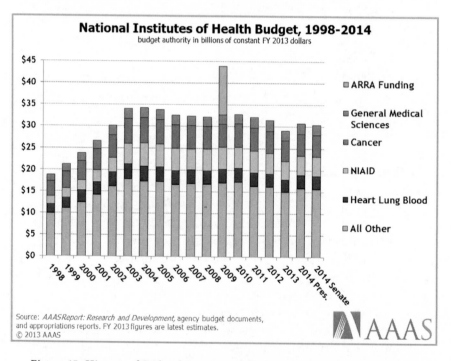

Figure 15. History of Federal Science Funding for the National Institutes of Health. Note large one year increase from the 2009 stimulus. The 2014 senate and presidential proposals for NIH funding are both quite close to $31B, but the house has proposed a 20 percent cut plus the sequester, arriving at around $24B. From AAAS Annual Report. http://www.aaas.org/spp/rd/Hist/Agencies.jpg.

The unpleasant reality is that there is no end in sight for the corrosive, destructive political battles that are gradually demolishing the scientific infrastructure of the U.S. Whereas the private sector may take up some of the slack, there is a limit to what it can contribute, both from the non-profits that focus on treatment for specific diseases, or from drug companies that are developing new therapies. In neither case do they prioritize the basic research needed for a thorough understanding and an answer to the questions posed above. The state governments are not much help either. While public and private universities have embarked upon a wild orgy of building construction in the last two decades, it is much easier to raise funds for university construction than to finance faculty salaries or fund research programs. During the last five decades, research funding has been looked upon as the responsibility of the federal government, and there is little interest contributing anymore than modest startup funds to the research programs of their faculty.

Another source of basic research discoveries were the private labs, funded by large, successful corporations. Yet these, too have declined or disappeared over the years. While Bell labs, RCA, Xerox, the Eastman labs, the Roche Institute and many other private labs over the years produced amazing discoveries and garnered their share of Nobel prizes, they have all but vanished from the American research scene.

Traditionally, university funds were given out in order to get young investigators going, the assumption being that they would be responsible for obtaining long term support through the NIH granting process. So the university support for new faculty members has usually been only for a four to five year period.

While overall support for scientific research continued to grow in the early years of this century, much of this was classified weapon research, sponsored by the Department of Defense. Already in the 1990s this grand bargain was breaking apart. In 1992–93, Congress cancelled funding for the supercollider, a huge particle accelerator, due to a combination of economic and political (but not scientific) reasons. This megascience project was underway in Texas, in an area south of Dallas, and at the time of the cancellation two billion dollars had already been expended. It was planned to open up a new world of discovery in high energy physics, and would have established United States leadership in the field for years to come. The focal point of particle physics research has now moved to CERN outside of Geneva, Switzerland, and leadership has been given to the European Union and will remain so for the foreseeable future.[2]

It is important to recognize that decisions that involve government and the scientific infrastructure are immense and virtually irreversible, like trying to change the course of the Titanic. It takes years and years to train personnel, to build facilities, acquire equipment, develop the plans for long term research projects that may stretch over decades or even the lifetimes of the personnel. Most critically, there is a culture surrounding different scientific disciplines. This can involve a whole network of hundreds or thousands of people who have built a tradition of working, talking, collaborating together over a period of years. They work together for decades, they train one another, they collaborate, they interact at all levels, they have mutual societies of trust, respect and understanding. They constitute a worldwide village. If these cities in the clouds are dismantled, they will not reappear in our lifetimes.

In the intervening years the sense has grown within the U.S. congress and in the public consciousness that science is simply not that important as a government function, and it is perfectly acceptable to surrender leadership to China,[3] the EU and a number of other Asian countries.

As I have indicated throughout this book, epigenetic research is on the cusp of an explosion today. There is a huge backlog of scientific projects that cannot move ahead because of a lack of funding. The most successful program for distribution of research dollars is the peer reviewed, individual investigator grant (known in the trade as the "RO 1 grant"). Yet every year the pressure ratchets up, as more investigators apply for a piece of an ever-shrinking budget (Figure 15).

Despite the tremendous excitement surrounding epigenetics today, it is increasingly difficult for individual scientists to obtain funding.[4] A proposal must pass through a gauntlet of skeptical reviewers, and councils that parcel out the funds. As budgets are cut over and over again, it becomes more and more difficult to carry on coherent, balanced, long term investigations. Investigators may be forced to plan from day to day, and lay off staff, damaging the stability of their programs.

"You Can't Solve Problems by Throwing Money at Them"

This is a refrain that we hear all the time from those who are unwilling to critically analyze government spending programs and separate things that work from things that don't work. If they were to do this, such critics would find that government funding for science has been an incredibly successful investment over the course of the last six decades, from 1945 up to the present.

Let's think about some of the more notable scientific achievements, brought about by government funding: The Hubble space telescope, the conquest of AIDS/HIV, the discovery of Prions (the cause of "mad cow disease"), the discovery of restriction enzymes (allowing genetic engineering to move forward), astronauts on the moon, the space station, polio vaccine, cracking the DNA code, discovery of oncogenes, spacecraft probes, witnessing Comet Shoemaker-Levy 9 smashing into Jupiter, discovery of alien planets, human embryonic stem cells, recovery of soft tissue from T. rex, the polymerase chain reaction, discovery of the different classes of RNA, discovery of DNA....

The list is practically endless. A feature that many of these discoveries (all supported partially or entirely by U.S. government funding) share is that they were long term programs that required years and years of reliable, continuous support, without any promise of payoff. There is no entity that can supply this kind of guarantee except the government.

Of all the advances that I have listed here, none can surpass the Curiosity landing on Mars for sheer audacity. Accomplished in 2012 after years of planning, the project required instrumentation of mind-boggling complexity, subject to blasts of radiation, extremes of temperature, zero vacuum, all required to work perfectly, millions of miles from Earth, with one and only one chance to get it right.[5]

15

The Way Forward

Epigenetics and Activism

In the 21st century, in an era of big everything, from cities to hamburgers to McMansions, it may seem that the individual has no power to influence outcomes that will affect his life and the lives of those around him. But there are actions that individuals and small groups take all the time, and some of these develop into powerful movements.

Probably the best example, relevant to the topic of this book, is the environmental movement that began as far back as the 1960s. Driven by the obvious effects of poor environmental stewardship, pressure from the American people on Congress during the 1960s and '70s resulted in the passage of a huge bundle of laws and the establishment of governmental bodies such as the EPA and the National Institute of Environmental Sciences for alleviating the effects of pollution and destruction of the environment. These accomplishments produced great benefits to the overall health and welfare of the American people and immense improvements in the quality of life. During this period average longevity increased and deaths from major illnesses declined.

But these accomplishments over the years may have built a sense of complacency in the American people, and certainly have fueled a powerful reaction on the part of the industrial sector. The result has been that laws are being reversed, benefits are being lost, and we are seeing disturbing and unexplained increases in the incidence of the epigenetically related illnesses described in these pages. Once again, a huge ship slowly turns about and reverses it course.

Why has the environmental movement stumbled and seemingly lost its ability to rally masses of enthusiastic supporters? It is startling to see the level of activism, the enthusiasm and the commitment of extremely conservative political action groups, especially at the local level. During the 1970s and 1980s I saw firsthand this activism, commitment and hard work completely reversed the politics of the state of Texas, from a state dominated by the Democratic Party to a state almost completely ruled by an extremely conservative Republican Party. These efforts have paid off for the conservative movement, even in states such as North Carolina and Wisconsin, nominally middle of the road "purple" states, but now completely dominated by conservative political agendas.

While environmentally conscious citizens may disagree with conservative political values, one must admire their success, and wonder how this level of energy might be directed toward confronting the issues raised by this book. Unfortunately this level of involvement at the so-called "grass roots" has not been seen in the environmental movement in decades; if it were today it would completely change the dynamics.

But You Can't Ban Everything

The realization that the epigenome is a fundamental part of our biology and a vital component of normal and diseased states provides understanding and guidance to a range of questions. The awareness that many artificial and naturally occurring substances may alter the organism's hereditary endowment can serve as a basis for responsible environmental stewardship. Furthermore, epigenetic changes can be monitored by following specific genetic regions and this can serve as a biomarker for disease and the response of the epigenome.

But if practically every diseased and normal state has an epigenetic component, doesn't this mean that in explaining everything we explain nothing? Isn't this situation similar to the genome searches, in which investigators turn up thousands of genes that play a role in IQ determination, but the contribution of each is so small that each bit of information provides little real knowledge? If so many natural and synthetic chemicals and so many stressful and traumatic events can produce changes in the epigenome, doesn't this face us with an impossible task? Where do you start? How can you concoct a reasonable, workable series of guidelines?

A serious consideration of epigenetics and its place in the world requires that we prioritize our needs. While there are thousands and thousands of chemicals and other possible epimutagenic substances, there are many whose effects are already widely recognized, are distributed throughout the environment, and could be controlled using existing technologies. These include the heavy metals and the most noxious organic compounds such as benzene. Anti regulatory folks will protest that these substances are already regulated (and perhaps shouldn't have been regulated in the first place). But that is hardly the point. An epigenetic analysis of the threat of these substances is essential. Decisions concerning "safe" levels in the environment were made years ago, and without any notion of the epigenetic landscape and how it affects the toxicity of these substances.

The Ames test was a useful test 40 years ago, based on the best science available at the time. But there are many new tests for epigenetic effects and they will need to be incorporated into environmental monitoring systems.[1]

Of course you can't ban everything, and at this stage in our understanding, this would be ruinous. Most of the substances that are burdened with epigenetic hazards were invented for very good reasons, and may have contributed greatly to a good quality of life in the 21st century. Removing them would require the introduction of substitutes which could be just as damaging, or worse. But this is a straw man argument.

I am asking for a recognition of the problem and an assurance on the part of our political establishment to investigate it. This commitment would require a reversal of the downward movement in funding for research and implementation of environmental monitoring; it's not going to break the bank, but it will cost billions.

What If I'm Wrong?

What if this whole volume is just a huge case of mistaken identity? What if epigenetics is really just a trivial sideline to the main message of hardwired genes and the genome? What if the essential picture that has dominated our thinking about heredity for the last century or more is really all there is? What if all the evidence that I have presented here, and the thousands and thousands of scientific papers on epigenetics that I have not presented[2] are in error, are poorly designed and executed, are misstatements, ignore critical factors? What if there are really no significant epigenetic hazards from the chemicals that squeeze themselves into every minute of every day of our lives? What if all the conventional explanations for these diseases and for their increase are correct and have nothing to do with epigenetics?

Perhaps autism is due entirely due to poor parenting, bad nutrition, DNA gene mutations. What if type II diabetes is simply the result of obesity and an excess of sugar that shuts down the insulin receptors? What if Alzheimer's disease is due to aluminum poisoning? Suppose bipolar disorder is simply due to lousy parenting? What if schizophrenia is due to hidden childhood trauma? What if all cancers are caused by viruses and bad genes and carcinogens that bust up DNA?

Well, I would respond that this outcome is so unlikely that it can be totally and irrevocably discounted, and denial of a mountain of epigenetic data would make an extremely poor basis for designing a long term healthcare strategy. The evidence for the epigenetic model is not incorrect or faulty. It is incomplete.

But if the epigenome model were simply wrong, and if we were guided by false information and insisted on a renewed and expanded biomedical investigation of epigenetics, what would be the damage? A revitalized program of biomedical research would fill in the holes in our understanding and what would emerge would be powerful predictive models of these diseases, even if it turned out that epigenetics were not a contributing factor.

If the epigenomic model were wrong or irrelevant, and we poured extraordinary resources into the biomedical sciences, we would recapture world leadership in the field, we would provide thousands and thousands of jobs for struggling scientists, we would supercharge the pharma companies to pursue new leads in drug discovery, we would enable universities to expand their educational mission, we would produce more sensible and economical environmental regulation and management.

And yes, we would spend billions and billions of dollars. And yes, money would be wasted and false leads and bad ideas would be pursued. But these diseases now cost hundreds and hundreds of billions of dollars and there no end in sight. There is no end to the human suffering and misery that comes from diseases that are light years away from our understanding. There is no deciding knowledge in sight. There are no cures in sight.[3]

What If Nothing Is Done?

What if, in spite of all these admonitions, the public does not take a role in the debate—what if politicians continue to do what they are doing or not doing? What if the existentialist terror of a budget shortfall overwhelms any desire on the part of the public to preserve the edifice of science in our country? What if budgets for basic scientific research continue to melt away every year at a rate of 1 or 2 or 5 or 30 percent?

If Americans continue to accept the status quo in political dialog, research at universities and governmental institutions will not cease overnight. The Chinese will not take the mantle of reigning science superpower from the United States tomorrow. Efforts to understand the connection between epimutagenic damage and the ascendancy of diseases thought to have an epigenetic basis will not grind to a halt. U.S. medical care will not drop below the level of that available in Mali.

Many countries throughout the world have strong research programs in basic medical sciences, and I can guarantee you that epigenetics will occupy a larger and larger part of their concerns. Perhaps the combined efforts of expanding commitments throughout the world and an atrophied but still functioning program in the United States will eventually bring a thorough consummation of the epigenetics revolution.

But it will be much slower, and it will not come in time to turn around the lives of millions of people already suffering from these diseases. It will certainly be an expensive decision, both in terms of dollars and in terms of human misery. Whether these diseases find their basis in an epigenetic mechanism or not, they will continue to increase in frequency until we understand them. We will no doubt see our total bill for medical care rise and we will see an increase in disabled individuals who are unable to function in society or as members of the work force.

I cannot find it within my heart to believe that this is the country in which most Americans want to live. We have the power to change this dismal scenario. But do we have the will to accomplish it? Since the origins of civilization 12,000 years ago there have been many societies that rose to challenges and prospered and many others that failed and were swept forever from the surface of the earth.

The coming years will reveal the answer.

Epilogue:
Concluding Thoughts
on the 40-Year-Old Mystery

It's been troubling me for the last four decades (well, I think about other stuff, too). I never did figure out why our cells were so unruly, why they were so unstable, why they mutated with such a high frequency. I don't work in a laboratory anymore, so I can't set up a whole new series of experiments, with all the great new tools that have been invented for studying epigenetics. As I indicated earlier, studies that took months or years to accomplish can now be carried out in days or weeks.

In going through the recent literature during the preparation of this book, I found several papers in which scientists had looked at the problem of epigenetic mutations in cultured cells, and using different systems from the one I used, had observed high frequencies of variation similar to what I had found.

So I can't say that my results were due to epigenetic variation, but their findings certainly fit what I was seeing.

I would be delighted to see someone else follow through on this fascinating question using the cells and systems that we were investigating.

Chapter Notes

Chapter 1

1. Business Standard. "It's all in the DNA." Accessed August 18, 2013. http://www.business-standard.com/article/management/it-s-all-in-the-dna-113081100604_1.html.

2. Lavoisier's famous contemporary, the mathematician Joseph-Louis Lagrange, remarked of this event, "It took them only an instant to cut off that head, and a hundred years may not produce another like it." Chemical Heritage foundation. "Lavoisier." http://www.chemheritage.org/discover/online-resources/chemistry-in-history/themes/early-chemistry-and-gases/lavoisier.aspx.

3. Today evolutionary biologists have entertained an alternative explanation: the giraffe's neck evolved through sexual selection, as males spar with their necks in competition for females. A longer and more powerful neck, well armored, allows males to achieve dominance during intrasexual combat. Size does matter. However, the "browsing in the trees" hypothesis still has its supporters. See Wilkinson DM, Ruxton GD. "Understanding selection for long necks in different taxa." *Biol Rev.* 2012;87(3):616–30.

4. The lack of a tangible physical mechanism that would give substance to a scientific hypothesis has long been a stumbling block to its acceptance. For years people suspected that DNA was the genetic material, but the models for its structure were so wrong-headed that there appeared to be no way that it could transmit heredity messages from one generation to another. Protein was widely ac-

cepted as the basic genetic material. Only a few pioneers (Watson and Crick) took the idea and ran with it early.

In a lighter vein, the scientific community has never taken extrasensory perception seriously, because there is no known mechanism by which thoughts can be transmitted over distance. We know for sure that we don't have radio transmitters in our heads, and no one has come up with a workable alternative. No matter how much anecdotal evidence its supporters come up with, until such a machine inside our heads is discovered, ESP will remain fringe science.

5. And maybe soon thereafter, $100 for a genome. CNN Money. "The race for the $100 genome." Accessed August 18, 2013. http://money.cnn.com/2013/06/25/technology/enterprise/low-cost-genome-sequencing/index.html. Genia Corporation website. Accessed August 18, 2013. http://www.geniachip.com/technology/.

6. Waddington CH. "The epigenotype: 1942." *Int J Epidemiol.* 2012;41(1):10–3.

7. The word "clone" comes from Greek, meaning "twig." Originally used in plant breeding, it refers to the fact that one can propagate many plants asexually, by rooting cutting from them. These cutting are (presumably) identical genetically to the original plant from which they were taken. In ordinary sexual reproduction egg and sperm are united and each generation represents a scrambling of the genetic input from two parents of the previous generation. In this fashion, new genetic combinations are generated in every generation, and old inferior ones are eliminated.

There are some very old clones in the world today. You might be a bit surprised to learn that stands of aspen trees are often clonal, growing from roots that spread out and form new trees. One clone of aspens in Colorado is said to be 80,000 years old. But as these clones age, they accumulate genetics damage and eventually the whole stand will become so debilitated that it will die out. This points out why sex is so important, if you didn't already know.
Ally D, Ritland K, Otto SP. "Aging in a long-lived clonal tree." *PLoS Biol.* 2010; 8(8).

8. Murphy SK, Jirtle RL. "Imprinting evolution and the price of silence." *Bioessays.* 2003;25(6):577–588.

9. Briggs R, King TJ. "Nuclear transplantation studies on the early gastrula (Rana pipiens) I. Nuclei of presumptive endoderm." *Dev Biol.* 1960;2(3):252–70.

10. Gurdon JB. "The cloning of a frog." *Development.* 2013;140(12):2446–8.

11. Hoppe PC, Illmensee K. "Full-term development after transplantation of parthenogenetic embryonic nuclei into fertilized mouse eggs." *Proc Natl Acad Sci U S A.* 1982;79(6):1912–6.

12. Cloning of farm animals has been thoroughly investigated and the FDA has concluded that it poses no risk. The report states in summary: "Because of their cost and rarity, clones will be used as any other specialized breeding stock are—to pass on naturally occurring, desirable traits such as disease resistance and higher quality meat to production herds. Almost all of the food that comes from the cloning process is expected to be from sexually reproduced descendants of clones, not the clones themselves." FDA. "Animal Cloning." Accessed August 20, 2013. http://www.fda.gov/Animal Veterinary/SafetyHealth/AnimalCloning/default.htm.

13. Normile D, Vogel G, Couzin J. "Cloning. South Korean team's remaining human stem cell claim demolished." *Science.* 2006;11(5758):156–7.

14. Oddly enough, it was later confirmed that one of Hwang's claims was authentic, the cloning of an afghan hound.

Experts who evaluated the evidence commented that this is especially bizarre, as cloning a dog is no doubt much more difficult than cloning a human. This is because the dog's reproductive cycle is complex, for reasons that we don't need to go into. Nonetheless the cloning of Snuppy (his *nom de clon*) has been established beyond a shadow of a doubt. The work was taken over by other Korean investigators, and now many healthy dogs have been obtained through this process.

15. The first time I sequenced a gene I used large gels to separate the parts, and it took days. Now you send it to a "core" facility at your university and it takes minutes.

16. Kuhn T. *The Structure of Scientific Revolutions.* Chicago: University of Chicago Press; 1962.

Chapter 2

1. This period was referred to as "The Golden Age of Molecular Biology" by Gunther Stent (1924–2008), a professor at the University of California. What Stent meant was that in this period the fundamental laws of life were discovered and elaborated upon; the nature of DNA, RNA and protein, the mechanisms by which information stored, saved, changed and acted upon in living systems. Stent, GS. *Molecular Genetics: An Introductory Narrative.* San Francisco: W.H. Freeman; 1971. Whereas our understanding of these processes had been greatly expanded upon during the intervening years, there will never be another period in which so many questions were answered by such a marvelous series of beautiful, logical and very simple experiments.

2. Invitrogen Corporation website. Accessed August 18, 2013. http://www.invitrogen.com/site/us/en/home/Products-and-Services/Applications/Sequencing/Next-Generation-Sequencing/ion-torrent-next-generation-sequencing-workflow/ion-torrent-next-generation-sequencing-run-sequence/ion-proton-system-for-next-generation-sequencing.html.

3. Scientific American blogs. Accessed August 19, 2013. http://blogs.scientific american.com/cross-check/2010/05/27/craig-venter-has-neither-created-nor-demystified-life/.

4. Cold Spring Harbor Laboratory website. Accessed August 18, 2013. http://www.dnalc.org/view/15073-Completion-of-a-draft-of-the-human-genome-Bill-Clinton.html.

5. In President Obama's January 2013 State of the Union address, he stated that the $3.8 billion investment in the human genome project had returned 141-fold the initial cost, yielding $800 billion in spinoff activities. I argued in *The Scientist* (http://www.the-scientist.com/?articles.view/articleNo/35680/title/Opinion—The-Payoff-of-Big-Science/) that the figure was grossly exaggerated. Obama's statement was based on a report from the Battelle Institute that appeared to factor in many advances in the life sciences that were made before the HGP was completed or were investigations that had little connection to it. Whereas the HGP was a fantastic technical *tour de force*, I don't believe that exaggerating its economic payback helps the cause of science.

6. The Marshall Protocol Knowledge Base. Accessed August 18, 2013. http://mpkb.org/home/alternate/genetic_predisposition.

7. *The Atlantic* website. Accessed October 6, 2013. http://www.theatlanticwire.com/technology/2010/08/genetic-scientist-we-have-learned-nothing-from-the-genome/19177/.

8. Throughout this book you will find a number of descriptions of different aspects of the molecular basis of epigenetics. Because of the primary focus of this book on medical, social, political and cultural issues, the descriptions of the complex mechanisms that make up the epigenetic machinery are kept to a minimum.

9. Yan C, Boyd DD. "Histone H3 acetylation and H3 K4 methylation define distinct chromatin regions permissive for transgene expression." *Mol Cell Biol.* 2006; 26(17):6357–71.

10. Davies K. "Encyclopedia Genomica: UK Scientists Print the Book of Life in 130 Volumes." *BioIT World.* December 28, 2012. Accessed August 13, 2013. http://www.bio-itworld.com/2012/12/28/encyclopedia-genomica-UK-scientists-print-book-of-life-in-130-volumes.html.

11. Nobel Prize Foundation website. Accessed August 19, 2013. http://www.nobelprize.org/nobel_prizes/medicine/laureates/1965/jacob-lecture.pdf.

12. Sadly, Jacob passed away at about the time of this writing.

13. Blumenthal T. "Operons in eukaryotes." *Brief Funct Genomic Proteomic.* (2004)3(3):199–211. This paper has a nice discussion of some recently uncovered operons in higher organisms. Yet as we will see, the really important account about control is the epigenetics story.

Chapter 3

1. http://famagusta-gazette.com/keijiro-matsushima-recalls-the-horror-of-hiroshima-p15557–69.htm.

2. There are, however, exceptions to the rule of genomic stability. For instance, on the Y chromosome (the chromosome that determines maleness), there are single bases (the familiar A, T, G, and C that make up the genetic code) that often vary from individual to individual (referred as SNPs) and can serve as road signs on the genetic map. They have mutation rates of 1 in a hundred million, a quite respectable figure. On the other hand, there are repeating segments of non-coding DNA that have mutation rates as high as one in a hundred. These markers on the Y chromosomes are used for studies of human ancestry, since the further two individuals are separated by their lineage, the greater the number of changes that will have occurred in their Y chromosomes during this intervening period. If you know how frequently these DNA marker change over time, you can estimate the number of years back to their common ancestor. See Bird SC. "Towards improvements in the estimation of the coalescent: implications for the most effective

use of Y chromosome short tandem repeat mutation rates." *PLoS One.* 2012;7(10). The different stability of different regions and sequences of DNA is no doubt due to proteins and other factors that recognize different three dimensional structures in the chromosomes and move in on them.

The incredible stability of a number of living creatures over geologic time is the result of a combination of a high level of stability for the genes that cause the organism's overall makeup, and the elimination by natural selection of any new, unfavorable mutations that do not improve the fitness or reproductive potential of the holder of these genes. Horseshoe crabs, ferns and cockroaches are so well adapted to their circumstances that improvements are very unlikely.

3. Carlson EA. "H.J. Muller's contributions to mutation research." *Mutat Res.* 2013. 752(1):1–5.

4. One of the most thoughtless and pernicious applications of X-rays, all but forgotten today, was the use of fluoroscopes in shoe stores during the 1930s and 40s. These devices were ubiquitous as a marketing tool; presumably to guarantee a perfect fit. You simply inserted your feet into the machine and you could wiggle your toes and see them move in the shoes that you were trying on. I clearly remember this experience, it was great fun. The problem was that X-ray machines were extremely inefficient in those times and sprayed huge doses of radiation around the store. The subject could receive 10 to 116 R in the space of 10 minutes. I tried to calculate the dose in modern terminology, and it appears that 100 R is something in the neighborhood of dose that many of the atomic bomb survivors received. This level of radiation caused burns and damage to the cartilage in the feet. The FDA banned the machines in 1953. See Nedd, CA, 2nd. "When the solution is the problem: a brief history of the shoe fluoroscope." *AJR Am J Roentgenol.* 1992;158(6):1270.

5. Adventurous as his life was, Muller could not have held a candle to his coworker and contemporary, Calvin Bridges, a pioneer of early 20th century genetics who discov-

ered the phenomenon of gene exchange in Drosophila. His life is the recent topic of a biopic, *The Fly Room,* made by geneticist Alexis Gambis, who began developing the idea for while working toward a Masters in film at New York University. "I focused on Calvin Bridges. He was this brilliant geneticist, but he was also bit of a James Dean type, who was known for being a womanizer." Bridges was known to frequent brothels and had several affairs. Bridges was light years away from the tell-alls of the Jerry Springer show and we will never know the details of his wild and brief life. Gambis states that when Bridges died of syphilis in 1938, his colleagues burned the notebook that contained his personal diaries in an attempt to protect his legacy. http://www.thescientist.com/?articles.view/articleNo/36594/title/A-Fly-on-the-Wall/.

6. General Accounting Office (GAO). Toxic Substances Control Act: Preliminary Observations on Legislative Changes to Make TSCA More Effective (Testimony, 07/13/94, GAO/T-RCED-94–263). Accessed August 21, 2013. http://www.gao.gov.

7. Brenner DJ, Hall EJ. "Computed tomography—an increasing source of radiation exposure." *N Engl J Med.* 2007; 357(22): 2277–84.

8. Lahav R. "Endothelin receptor B is required for the expansion of melanocyte precursors and malignant melanoma." *Int J Dev Biol.* 2005;49(2–3):173–80.

9. Kurttio P, et al. "Fallout from the Chernobyl accident and overall cancer incidence in Finland." *Cancer Epidemiol.* 2013;7(5):585–92.

10. Ogrodnik A, Hudon TW, Nadkarni PM, Chandawarkar RY. "Radiation exposure and breast cancer: lessons from Chernobyl." *Conn Med.* 2013;77(4):227–34.

11. Many of the observations of the area around Chernobyl in the years following the accident appear counterintuitive. Because a large section of the region is cordoned off and the entire human population was moved out by the Soviet government, there has been an upsurge in the wildlife and plant populations. Many species that were absent from this region, such as

wolves, have returned. See Yablokov AV. "Chernobyl's radioactive impact on fauna." *Ann N Y Acad Sci.* 2009;1181:255–80. Radiation levels in this zone of exclusion are still so high that workers continuing remediation on the reactor are only permitted to work five hours a day for one month before taking 15 days of rest. Governmental officials estimate the area will not be safe for human populations for another 20,000 years. I recommend to the reader many of the fine documentaries that have been filmed describing the aftermath of the disaster. A beautiful and evocative *Nature* documentary was filmed in 2011 and portrays the stunning post-apocalypse appearance of the area, and the profusion of wildlife. http://www.pbs.org/wnet/nature/episodes/radioactive-wolves/full-episode/7190/. Written reports simply do not convey the emotional impact of these events.

12. McCarrey and his colleagues have published some very interesting studies in which they show that the germ line (those cells that produce the eggs and sperm for the next generation) are more stable than the somatic cells (the rest of the body cells) that will not pass on their genes to subsequent generations). This makes sense from an evolutionary standpoint; species that minimize their genetic mistakes will produce less debilitated offspring. "It is particularly important for genetic integrity to be maintained in these cells and therefore relatively beneficial for germ cells to exert additional energy to achieve this." See McCarrey JR. "The epigenome as a target for heritable environmental disruptions of cellular function." *Mol Cell Endocrin.* 2012; 354(1–2):9–15. This repair also applies to some epigenetic mutations.

Chapter 4

1. Today cell culture is universally performed with plastic culture flasks, and the liquid media used are prepared and stored in plastic containers. The media are transferred using plastic tubing and disposable plastic pipettes. Unfortunately, plasticizers and other molecules can leach into the media. This means that if you are testing certain chemicals for their effects on cells in culture, you are not starting from zero, as the cells may already be exposed to chemicals similar to the ones you are examining. Furthermore, plastic storage materials are universally employed in the medical industry, and the effects of phthalates and other material leaching into medicinal solutions is unknown. This shows how widespread these substances are, if we have to struggle just to find an uncontaminated control series. There is already a substantial peer-reviewed literature on this topic. See for example Latini G, Ferri M, Chiellini F. "Materials degradation in PVC medical devices, DEHP leaching and neonatal outcomes." *Curr Med Chem.* 2010;17(26):2979–89.

2. When reports of birth defects from thalidomide began appearing, the manufacturer, Chemie Grünenthal, found that an obscure breed, the White New Zealand rabbit, also gave birth to malformed offspring, but only at a dose between 25 to 300 times that given to humans (*Exp Mol Path Supl.* 1963;2:81–106; *Federation Proceedings.* 1967;26:1131–6; *Teratogenesis, Carcinogenesis, and Mutagenesis* 1982;2:361–74). "Safer Medicines." Accessed August 23, 2103. http://www.safermedicines.org/faqs/faq17.shtml.

3. Carlsson HE, Schapiro SJ, Farah I, Hau J. "Use of primates in research: a global overview." *Am J Primatol.* 2004;63(4):225–37. The paper states that "a total of 2,937 articles involving 4,411 studies that employed nonhuman primates or nonhuman primate biological material were identified and analyzed. More than 41,000 animals were represented in the studies published in 2001."

4. As our understanding of animal intelligence has expanded, the ethical issues of animal experimentation loom larger. Philosophers and scientists from Descarte to B. F.Skinner looked upon animals as machines, automatons, unable to experience pain or any other human emotion. Studies attempting to measure animal IQ were so primitive that the generally accepted mantra was that "animal cognition" was an oxymoron, and only humans were capable of complex patterns of reasoning. It turns

out that the lack of intelligence was in the scientists, not the animals they were studying. Much more sophisticated testing reveals that not only primates but many other mammals are able to manipulate tools, cooperate for an imagined goal, display generosity and sharing, and even, in the case of elephants, morn their dead. For centuries pet owners have been accused of anthropomorphizing displays of animal brilliance, but many such claims can be replicated in the laboratory, provided the investigators are sufficiently imaginative. Such observations have caused animal care and use committees to become more and more restrictive over the years with regard to acceptable experimental procedures. See "The Brains of the Animal Kingdom." *Wall Street Journal*. Accessed August 21, 2103. http://online.wsj.com/article/SB 10001424127887323869604578370574285382756.html.

Another fascinating study described how dogs were trained to remain immobile in an MRI machine so that investigator could study their brain function while they were alert and unanaesthetized. The results demonstrate that dogs have rich and varied neuronal activity, comparable to young human children. See Berns G. "Dogs *are people too.*" *New York Times, October 15, 2013. http://www.nytimes.com/2013/10/06/opinion/sunday/dogs-are-people-too.html?_r=1&adxnnl=1&pagewanted=2&adxnnlx=1381848759-BBfnJkQRf7+ipaZUWRm73g&single=1.*

5. Strasak AM, et al. "Statistical errors in medical research—a review of common pitfalls." Swiss Med Wkly. 2007;137(3-4):44–9. Unfortunately, you can plug your data into many different statistical programs that you can download from the Internet. But if you haven't vetted your analysis with a good biostatistician, you can arrive at answers that are wildly inappropriate.

6. "Cancer Research UK." Accessed August 23, 2013. http://www.cancerresearchuk.org/cancer-info/news/archive/press release/2010-07-12-deadly-cancer-survival-doubles.

Chapter 5

1. Archigenes of Apamea, a Roman medical practitioner, practiced state of the art cancer surgery. He notes that any part of the human body should be removed surgically when affected by sepsis or by certain types of carcinoma, because these parts have already lost their natural connection to the body. Then, he stresses the importance of early diagnosis, because at such a stage, the carcinoma may be healed with the aid of medicaments, avoiding surgery. If, nevertheless, cancer is diagnosed in an advanced stage, excision of the growth is absolutely necessary, although only if the patient is strong and has power to cope with the operation. For more fascinating details check Papavramidou, N, Papavramidis, T, and Demetriou, T. "Ancient Greek and Greco–Roman methods in modern surgical treatment of cancer." *Ann Surg Oncol.* 2010;17(3): 665–7.

An interesting glance at medieval medicine: "The history of surgery in the middle ages is a surprisingly progressive one, thanks largely to experience gained by the butcher-surgeons on the battle field and due to natural and herbal medicines such as mandrake root, hemlock and opium, which were used as anesthetics and wine which was used as an antiseptic. In the thirteenth century, Theodoric Lucca wrote: 'Every day we see new instruments and new methods [of removing arrows from wounded soldiers] being invented by clever and ingenious surgeons.'"

It seems that medical science has always had its cheerleaders. "Articles on History." Accessed August 23, 2013. http://www.articlesonhistory.com/medieval-medicine.php.

2. Cancer.org. Accessed August 18, 2013. http://www.cancer.org/research/cancerfacts statistics/cancerfactsfigures2013/index.

3. Cat fanciers are familiar with the feline leukemia virus, for which an effective vaccine is available.

4. Internet Media Center. Accessed August 18, 2013. http://www.who.int/media centre/factsheets/fs297/en/.

5. Reuters. Accessed August 18, 2013.

http://www.reuters.com/article/2012/10/11/us-drugs-dendreon-provenge-idUSBRE89A15420121011.

6. Shore ND, et al. "Building on sipuleucel-T for immunologic treatment of castration-resistant prostate cancer." *Cancer Control.* 2013;20(1):7–16.

7. Wurz GT, et al. "Antitumor effects of L-BLP25 Antigen-Specific tumor immunotherapy in a novel human MUC1 transgenic lung cancer mouse model." *J Transl Med.* 2013;11(1):64.

8. Bota, S., et al. "Follow-up of bronchial precancerous lesions and carcinoma *in situ* using fluorescence endoscopy." *Am J Respir Crit Care Med.* 2001; 164(9):1688–93.

9. "Questionable methods of cancer management: Electronic devices." *CA Cancer J Clin.* 1994;44(12):115–27.

10. Probably one of the saddest stories of phony cancer treatments concerns the tough guy movie actor Steve McQueen, who was diagnosed with mesothelioma, from which he died in 1980. McQueen was a heavy smoker and had worked around asbestos in ship building yards as a kid. McQueen underwent a quack treatment in Mexico with the drug Laetrile, which had never been approved by the FDA. Although he initially claimed he was cured, he died a few months later. His physician, Dr. William D. Kelley, was blacklisted by the American Cancer Society. http://www.nytimes.com/2005/11/15/health/15essa.html?_r=0.

11. For example, "Richard Nixon launched the so-called War on Cancer on December 23, 1971, in what was supposed to be a 'moonshot' effort to cure the disease. Two years later, a *Time* magazine cover read, 'Toward Control of Cancer.' Two decades after that, it announced, in bold red letters, 'Hope in the War Against Cancer,' surmising that 'a turning point' may have been reached. In 2001, its cover asked if the blood cancer drug Gleevec 'is the breakthrough we've been waiting for.' And this past April, the newsweekly pronounced 'How to Cure Cancer.'" "World War Cancer." Accessed August 23, 2013, http://www.newyorker.com/online/blogs/elements/2013/07/world-war-cancer.html.

12. "Herceptin extends life of patients with terminal stomach cancer, study finds." Accessed Auguse 23, 2013. http://phys.org/news163089110.html.

13. "American Cancer Society Statistics." Accessed August 23, 2013, http://www.cancer.org/research/cancerfactsstatistics/.

14. "Nobel Prizes.org" Accessed August 23, 2013. http://www.nobelprize.org/nobel_prizes/medicine/laureates/1989/press.html.

15. A classic example of an oncogene that blocks cancer is the gene for retinoblastoma, a tumor of the retina of the eye. Ordinarily, the gene produces an inhibitor of cancerous growth, but when it mutates, is loses its preventive properties and growth is unhinged. Sage J. "The retinoblastoma tumor suppressor and stem cell biology." *Genes Dev.* 2012;26(13):1409–20.

16. Ujvari B, et al. "Evolution of a contagious cancer: epigenetic variation in Devil Facial Tumour Disease." *Proc Biol Sci.* 2013;280(1750):20121720.

17. Copeland RA, Moyer MP, Richon VM. "Targeting genetic alterations in protein methyltransferases for personalized cancer therapeutics." *Oncogene.* 2013;32 (8):939–46.

18. Seow WJ, et al. "Urinary benzene biomarkers and DNA methylation in Bulgarian petrochemical workers: study findings and comparison of linear and beta regression models." *PLoS One.* 2012;7(12): e504.

19. Zöchbauer-Müller S, Minna JD, Gazdar AF. "Aberrant DNA methylation in lung cancer: biological and clinical implications." *Oncologist.* 2002;7(5):451–7.

20. The lethal effects of smoking are now so widely acknowledged that the tobacco companies are using it as a marketing tool. In 2000 Philip Morris commissioned Arthur D. Little to do a study comparing the health costs of treating patient with smoking-related diseases with the cost savings due to their premature death, which would lower social security costs. It was found that smokers saved the government money, because they die so young

that their healthcare costs are offset by their inability to collect social security. The study was to be used as a marketing tool to convince the Czech government that it would not be in their best interests to run anti-smoking campaigns. After an extremely animated executive session at their European headquarters in Neuchatel, Switzerland (a non-smoking facility), it was decided not to push the results of the study. It was argued successfully that the public would perceive the cigarette industry as heartless. Nonetheless the study was widely denigrated as an attempt to do away with old people. Philip Morris vigorously denied this characterization, stating that it was merely an economic analysis for informational purposes. Dembart L. "Tobacco Giant's Analysis Says Premature Deaths Cut Costs in Pensions and Health Care: Critics Assail Philip Morris Report on Smoking." *The New York Times.* July 18, 2001. http://www.nytimes.com/2001/07/18/news/18iht-smoking_ed3_.html.

21. Singh S, Li SS. "Epigenetic effects of environmental chemicals bisphenol a and phthalates." *Int J Mol Sci.* 2012;13(8):10143–53.

22. "Asbestos and the World Trade Center." Accessed August 23, 2013. http://www.asbestos.com/world-trade-center/.

23. Daubriac JD, et al. "Molecular changes in mesothelioma with an impact on prognosis and treatment." *Arch Pathol Lab Med.* 2012;136(3):277–93.

24. Forsberg PA, Mark TM. "Pomalidomide in the treatment of relapsed multiple myeloma." *Future Oncol.* 2013;9(7):939–48.

25. Zhang X, et al. "Genome-wide study of DNA methylation alterations in response to diazinon exposure in vitro." *Environ Toxicol Pharmacol.* 2012;34(3):959–68.

26. Walker CL, Ho SM. "Developmental reprogramming of cancer susceptibility." *Nat Rev Cancer.* 2012;12(7):479–86.

Chapter 6

1. Sanghera DK, Blackett PR. "Type 2 diabetes genetics: Beyond GWAS." *J Diabetes Metab.* 2013;3(198).

2. Thayer KA, et al. "Role of environmental chemicals in diabetes and obesity: a National Toxicology Program workshop review." *Environ Health Perspect.* 2012;120 (6):779–89.

3. One of the most frequently asked questions regarding diabetes and diet is "Can diabetics drink alcohol?" The answer is a qualified "Yes"; moderate use with food, no sugary cocktails, one drink per day. "Diabetes WebMD." Accessed August 25, 2013. http://diabetes.webmd.com/drinking-alcohol.

4. Nikoshkov A, et al. "Epigenetic DNA methylation in the promoters of the Igf1 receptor and insulin receptor genes in db/db mice." *Epigenetics.* 2011;6(4):405–9.

5. Ling C, Groop L. "Epigenetics: a molecular link between environmental factors and type 2 diabetes." *Diabetes.* 2009;58 (12):2718–25.

6. One of the great tools of modern molecular biology was the discovery and development of the green fluorescent protein. Isolated from a jellyfish, the gene specifying the protein has been transferred into many different species. When irradiated with ultraviolet light it gives off a ghostly green color, so it can be used as a marker for gene expression. It has the source of thousands of papers studying gene expression in a wide range of species and it has proved invaluable for following gene activity. Because the zebra fish is transparent, the combination of these tools is ideal for innumerable investigations. See "How a jellyfish protein transformed science." Accessed August 25, 2013. http://www.livescience.com/16752-gfp-protein-fluorescent-nih-nigms.html.

7. Moss JB, et al. "Regeneration of the pancreas in adult zebrafish." *Diabetes.* 2009;58(8):1844–51.

8. Vrachnis N, et al. "Impact of maternal diabetes on epigenetic modifications leading to diseases in the offspring." *Exp Diabetes Res.* 2012:538474.

9. There is an organization, the Caloric Restriction Society, that argues that lowering caloric intake drastically will improve health and longevity. There is a lot of con-

flicting evidence on this issue, so I don't recommend it to you at this time. In a country where obesity is an overwhelming problem, it is certainly in no danger of taking over the eating habits of the American public. "The Caloric Restriction Society." Accessed September 3, 2013. http://www.crsociety.org/.

10. Harith HH, Morris MJ, Kavurma MM. "On the TRAIL of obesity and diabetes." *Trends Endocrinol Metab.* 2013;24 (11):578–87.

11. Schulz L. "The Dutch hunger winter and the developmental origins of health and disease." *Proc Natl Acad Sci U S A.* 2010;107(39):16757–58.

12. Meymandi, A. "The science of epigenetics." *Psychiatry (Edgmont).* 2010;7(3): 40–41.

13. Nitert MD, et al. "Impact of an exercise intervention on DNA methylation in skeletal muscle from first-degree relatives of patients with type 2 diabetes." *Diabetes.* 2012;61(12):3322–32.

14. Morbidity and Mortality Weekly Report (MMWR). "Increasing Prevalence of Diagnosed Diabetes-United States and Puerto Rico, 1995–2010." http://www.cdc.gov/mmwr/preview/mmwrhtml/mm61 45a4.htm.

15. "Eat Like a Mennonite." Accessed August 25, 2013. http://www.nytimes.com/2013/01/19/opinion/eat-like-a-mennonite.html?_r=0 .

16. Wei, J, et al. "Perinatal exposure to bisphenol A at reference dose predisposes offspring to metabolic syndrome in adult rats on a high-fat diet." *Endocrinology.* 2011; 152(8):3049–61.

17. Dolinoy DC, Huang D, Jirtle RL. "Maternal nutrient supplementation counteracts bisphenol A-induced DNA hypomethylation in early development." *Proc Natl Acad Sci U S A.* 2007;104(42):13056–61.

18. Shankar A, Teppala S, Sabanayagam C. "Bisphenol A and peripheral arterial disease: results from the NHANES." *Environ Health Perspect.* 2012;120(9):1297–1300.

19. Kim K, Park H. "Association between urinary concentrations of bisphenol A and type 2 diabetes in Korean adults: a population-based cross-sectional study." *Int J Hyg Environ Health.* 2013;216(4):467–71.

20. "The Endocrine Society Supports FDA Science Board's Actions On Bisphenol A." Accessed August 25, 2013. https://www.endocrine.org/news-room/press-release-archives/2008/103108bpanewsrelease.

Chapter 7

1. Quiroga, PQ, Fried, I, Koch C. "Brain cells for grandmother." *Sci Am.* 2013; 308 (2):31–5.

2. Some years ago I was with a group of colleagues from my university at a conference in Cuernavaca, Mexico. One evening we visited a nightclub to hear a Beatles tribute band. They had an extensive repertoire, covering virtually all of the Beatles songs. During their break I attempted to engage the leader of the group in conversation. I was astonished to find that none of them spoke a word of English, even though they had memorized dozens of Beatles songs. A formidable display of memory!

3. Alzheimer's Disease International. "World Alzheimer Report 2010: The global economic impact of dementia. 2010." Accessed August 23, 2013. http://www.alz.co.uk/research/files/WorldAlzheimer-Report2010.pdf

4. Tejada-Vera B. "Mortality From Alzheimer's Disease in the United States: Data for 2000 and 2010. NCHS Data Brief #116. March 2013."

5. See "Alzheimer's treatment failed trial, maker says." Accessed August 26, 2013. http://www.nytimes.com/2013/05/08/business/baxter-says-its-new-alzheimers-treatment-has-failed.html?_r=0, for a detailed discussion of this problem.

6. Kim S., et al. "The preventive and therapeutic effects of intravenous human adipose-derived stem cells in Alzheimer's disease mice." *PLoS One.* 2012;7(9):1–17.

At present there are no stem cell therapies approved by the FDA. There are many foreign clinics that claim success in the treatment of many diseases, but these are basically scams, charging huge sums for unproven, ineffective and dangerous procedures.

7. The GWAS approach is highly controversial. If you Google "failure of GWAS" you will find many articles that highlight the debate between experts.

8. Golde TE, et al. "Alzheimer's disease risk alleles in TREM2 illuminate innate immunity in Alzheimer's disease." *Alzheimers Res Ther.* 2013;5(3):24.

9. Stiller JW, Weinberger DR. "Boxing and chronic brain damage." *Psychiatr Clin North Am.* 1985;8(2):339–56.

10. Cook, K. "Dying to Play." *New York Times,* September 11, 2012. Accessed August 23, 2013. http://www.nytimes.com/2012/09/12/opinion/head-injuries-in-football.html?.

11. Corcellis J, et al. "The aftermath of boxing." *Psychol Med.* 1973;3(3):270–303; Kelland K. "Should science on brain injury inspire a ban on boxing?" Accessed August 26, 2013, http://www.reuters.com/article/2013/03/21/us-boxing-brain-idUSBRE92K03720130321.

12. Gu Y, Scarmeas N. "Dietary patterns in Alzheimer's disease and cognitive aging." *Curr Alzheimer Res.* 2011;8(5):510–9.

There is an increasing body of evidence that taking vitamin and mineral supplements on top of a normal, healthy diet is a serious health risk. There is no evidence that increasing vitamin and mineral levels over the known optimum will improve health. See http://www.theatlantic.com/health/archive/2011/11/are-supplements-killing-you-the-problem-with-vitamins-minerals/248450/.

13 Mikaelsson MA, Miller CA. "DNA methylation: a transcriptional mechanism co-opted by the developed mammalian brain?" *Epigenetics.* 2011;6(5):548–51. In this largely speculative and theoretical article the authors present data based on a fear conditioning paradigm. Rats are given a mild foot shock and changes in the DNA of cells in the cells of the hippocampus are followed. The authors state, "Specifically, methylation levels of the memory-enhancing gene, *reelin,* decreased. Simultaneously, methylation of the memory-

suppressing gene, *PP1,* increased. Both genes demonstrated transcription changes that corresponded to the transcriptional repression associated with DNA methylation. Importantly, these learning-induced methylation changes were prevented by DNA methyl transferase inhibition at the time of training and returned to basal levels with 24 h."

Our understanding of memory and learning is still in its infancy, but the authors conclude their observations by stating, "Collectively, these studies provide compelling evidence for the involvement of DNA methylation in learning and memory. (They) also suggest that DNA methylation can provide an organism with a dynamic mode to regulate transcription of genes important to memory function during the earlier period of synaptic consolidation, (and) serving as a more stable epigenetic marker during system consolidation. One question lurking on the horizon: What mechanisms are employed by the CNS to regulate these qualitatively different modes of DNA methylation?"

14. Ferreira PC, Piai Kde A, Takayanagui AM, Segura-Muñoz SI. "Aluminum as a risk factor for Alzheimer's disease." *Rev Lat Am Enfermagem.* 2008;16(1):151–7.

15. Bakulski KM, Rozek LS, Dolinoy DC, Paulson HL, Hu H. "Alzheimer's disease and environmental exposure to lead: the epidemiologic evidence and potential role of epigenetics." *Curr Alzheimer Res.* 2012;9(5):563–73. This is an especially good paper, with lots of information on all aspects of Alzheimer's and epigenetics.

16. Bakulski KM, et al. "Genome-wide DNA methylation differences between late-onset Alzheimer's disease and cognitively normal controls in human frontal cortex." *J Alzheimers Dis.* 2012;29(3):571–88.

17. Rao JS, Keleshian VL, Klein S, Rapoport SI. "Epigenetic modifications in frontal cortex from Alzheimer's disease and bipolar disorder patients." *Transl Psychiatry.* 2012;2.

18. Konsoula Z, Barile FA. "Epigenetic histone acetylation and deacetylation mechanisms in experimental models of neurode-

generative disorders." *J Pharmacol Toxicol Methods.* 2012;66(3):215–20.

19. Gräff J, et al. "An epigenetic blockade of cognitive functions in the neurodegenerating brain." *Nature.* 2012; 483(7388):222–6.

The authors point out that their results may explain why in some clinical trials, there is no improvement in function in Alzheimer's patients despite successful clearance of the amyloid proteins. They argue that once the epigenetic blockade is in place, reducing amyloid protein production and deposition may not be sufficient to rescue cognitive function.

They propose a dual approach, by which amyloid reduction is combined with inhibition of HDAC2. By extension, these findings pinpoint HDAC2 as the likely target of nonselective HDAC inhibitors that counteract cognitive decline in AD mouse models and, as a result, strongly advocate for the development of HDAC2-selective inhibitors. Finally, the authors believe that their observations that HDAC2 inhibition likely re-instates function in the surviving neurons of the neurodegenerating brain raises hope that such plasticity is not irrevocably lost, but merely constrained by the epigenetic blockade.

20. Karagiannis TC and Ververis K. "Potential of chromatin modifying compounds for the treatment of Alzheimer's disease." *Pathobiol Aging Age Relat Dis.* 2012;2(10).

21. See "World Health Rankings." Accessed August 26, 2013. http://www.worldlifeexpectancy.com/cause-of-death/alzheimers-dementia/by-country/.

22. "Yale Environment 360: What Makes Europe Greener than the U.S.?" Accessed September 1, 2013. http://e360.yale.edu/feature/what_makes_europe_greener_than_the_us/2193/.

23. Brewer GJ. "The risks of copper toxicity contributing to cognitive decline in the aging population and to Alzheimer's disease." *J Am Coll Nutr.* 2009;28(3):238–42.

24. Dyer C. "Flu vaccine investigator is suspended for four months for research fraud." *BMJ.* 2012;16.

25. Cribbs DH. "Abeta DNA vaccination for Alzheimer's disease: focus on disease prevention." *CNS Neurol Disord Drug Targets.* 2010;9(2):207–16.

Chapter 8

1. NHLB Institute. "What is hemophilia?" http://www.nhlbi.nih.gov/health/health-topics/topics/hemophilia/.

2. A history of the eugenics movement is way beyond the scope of this book, and would constitute a heavy volume in its own right. In fact, there are a number excellent studies that have been written on this topic. The one that I used in my teaching was *In the Name of Eugenics: Genetics and the Uses of Human Heredity,* by Daniel Jo Kevles, Harvard University Press, 1998. The author discusses in detail the fact that American geneticists used twin study data in the 1920s and 1930s to provide an intellectual justification of genetic inferiority of races and classes. These studies were used by politicians to promote programs of sterilization of what they considered "inferior genotypes." Their data was lauded and employed by German university professors in the 1930 when they laid the "scientific" foundations of what would become the holocaust. They were highly regarded by the Nazi authorities, and received promotions, professorships and research grants to promote their studies. After the war, most continued their careers, which were long and successful, in a reconstructed Democratic West Germany.

The genetic basis of the variation in intelligence in human populations has been notoriously difficult to document. Many problematic studies were carried out in the second half of the 20th century using the twin study method, and were used to justify a questionable conservative social agenda. Arthur Jensen, a highly controversial social psychologist, argued that there were innate differences in IQ between blacks and whites that were most likely due to genetic factors. In fact, one of his arguments was that Head Start and other programs designed to boost the scholastic performance of minorities were bound to fail, because 80 percent of the variance in IQ scores was the result of genetic factors and only 20 percent could ascribed to environmental influences.

Today it is generally accepted that the variation in intelligence that we see in human populations is due in part to many different gene forms or alleles, perhaps hundreds or thousands. Each single gene makes only a tiny contribution to the overall makeup or phenotype of the individual. The relative contribution of genes and environments to intellectual performance is still unknown.

3. Lewis DA, Sweet RA. "Schizophrenia from a neural circuitry perspective: advancing toward rational pharmacological therapies." *J Clin Invest.* 2009;119(4):706–16.

4. Insel TR, Wang PS. "The STAR*D trial: revealing the need for better treatments." *Psychiatr Serv.* 2009;60(11):1466–7.

5. Rao JS, Keleshian VL, Klein S, Rapoport SI. "Epigenetic modifications in frontal cortex from Alzheimer's disease and bipolar disorder patients." *Transl Psychiatry.* 2012;2.

6. Bohacek J, Mansuy IM. "Epigenetic inheritance of disease and disease risk." *Neuropsychopharmacology.* 2013;38(1):220–36. This is an excellent review that brings together a lot of the evidence for environmental influence on epigenetic changes in genes that affect expression of normal and pathological brain function. There is an interesting passage that demonstrates the commitment that scientists show to their profession: "Brain functions generally benefit from stimulating environmental conditions, a concept that was initially demonstrated experimentally by Donald Hebb in 1947. He reported that rats that were raised free-roaming in his house outperformed rats raised in cages on problem-solving tasks." It is not reported how Mrs. Hebb dealt with this experimental protocol.

7. "Severe Psychiatric Disorders May Be Increasing." Accessed August 26, 2013. http://www.schizophrenia.com/newsletter/allnews/2002/disordersincrease.htm.

8. Peter CJ, Akbarian S. "Balancing histone methylation activities in psychiatric disorders." *Trends in Mol Med.* 2011;17 (7):372–79.

9. Hoek HW, et al. "Schizoid personality disorder after prenatal exposure to famine." *Am J Psychiatry.* 1996;153(12):1637–39.

10. Kirkbride JB, et al. "Prenatal nutrition, epigenetics and schizophrenia risk: can we test causal effects?" *Epigenomics.* 2012;4(3):303–15.

11. St. Clair D, Xu M, Wang P, et al. "Rates of adult schizophrenia following prenatal exposure to the Chinese famine of 1959–1961." *JAMA* 2005;294(5):557–62.

12. There has been much yammering over the years blaming ergot poisoning for the Salem witch trials. Ergot is a fungus that contaminates bread, and its ingestion can bring on convulsions and spasms. It has been suggested on many occasions that an epidemic of ergot poisoning brought on the bizarre behavior of the women who were accused of witchcraft. However, a careful analysis of reports taken at the time of the event show that the symptoms displayed were nothing like ergot poisoning and the events are better attributed to mass hysteria and a breakdown of the flimsy social fabric of the time. See Spanos NP, Gottlieb J. "Ergotism and the Salem Village witch trials." *Science.* 1976;194(4274):1390–4. These events were used by Arthur Miller in his play *The Crucible* as an analogy of the anti-communist witch hunts of the 1950s. Miller got it right, as he always did.

13. Gos M. "Epigenetic mechanisms of gene expression regulation in neurological diseases." *Acta Neurobiol Exp (Wars).* 2013;73(1):19–37.

Chapter 9

1. "NIH Autism Fact Sheet." http://www.ninds.nih.gov/disorders/autism/detail_autism.htm

2. CDC website. "Autism Spectrum Disorder." Accessed August 27, 2013. http://www.cdc.gov/ncbddd/autism/data.html.

3. In discussing the diagnosis (or over-diagnosis) with Emily Williams, she added some interesting perspectives:

For my part, I don't necessarily think over-diagnosis is an issue as much as good diagnosis. Being a good diagnostician and really understanding the cognitive roots of autism, as opposed to reviewing a checklist of behaviors, requires a special capacity by the professional—which many don't have. Akin to finding a talented teacher, a great therapist, or an excellent doctor. It's an art.

I think that a minority of the human spectrum will exhibit this constellation of traits, some of whom will fall very obviously into the "disordered" range, meanwhile others will display subtler deficits. [An acquaintance of mine] received an Asperger's diagnosis years ago, and while it may've been more believable then, [their] present social difficulties are not significant. However, certain learning deficits still provide (substantial) challenges.

I have come to believe that the symptoms known as "autism" are much more prevalent than was once believed, and can occur in both severely disabling and (relatively) minor forms. The latter may be the equivalent severity of something like ADHD, which may provide a better analogy. I have concluded that our labels are still in a state of adaptation to the reality of the human spectrum. There are those professionals who would disagree and state emphatically that all forms of autism must be severely disabling. But I simply ask "Why?" It seems that such opinions are based on belief rather than observation. If one would observe many of those who are extremely high-functioning, they would see that the challenges, though comparatively less, are quite similar.

4. Faras H, Al Ateeqi N, Tidmarsh L. "Autism spectrum disorders." *Ann Saudi Med.* 2010;30(4):295–300.

5. Frances A. *Saving Normal: An Insider's Revolt Against Out-of-Control Psychiatric Diagnosis, DSM-5, Big Pharma, and the Medicalization of Ordinary Life.* New York: William Morrow; 2013.

6. Buxhoeveden DP, Casanova MF. "The minicolumn hypothesis in neuroscience." *Brain.* 2002;125(Pt 5):935–51.

7. "The blue brain project." Accessed August 27, 2013. http://bluebrain.epfl.ch/page-89583-en.html. The website contains enthusiastic reports on progress: "Blue Brain is a resounding success. In five years of work, Henry Markram's team has perfected a facility that can create realistic models of one of the brain's essential building blocks. This process is entirely data driven and essentially automatically executed on the supercomputer. Meanwhile the generated models show a behavior already observed in years of neuroscientific experiments. These models will be basic building blocks for larger scale models leading towards a complete virtual brain." There does appear to be quite an overlap with the U.S. effort, now being pushed by the Obama administration.

8. "Allen Brain atlas." Accessed September 1, 2013. http://www.brain-map.org/.

9. "President Obama's brain map project is hardly the next Human Genome: The BRAIN research initiative is a big dream with a hefty price tag. That money would be better spent on other science research." Accessed August 27, 2013. http://www.theguardian.com/commentisfree/2013/apr/02/president-obama-brain-mapping-project-not-ideal.

10. Mameza MG, et al. "SHANK3 mutations associated with autism facilitate ligand binding to the Shank3 Ankyrin repeat region." *J Biol Chem.* 2013;288(37):26697–708.

11. "DNA learning center: autism candidate genes." Accessed September 1, 2013. http://www.dnalc.org/view/908-Autism-Candidate-Genes.html.

12. Winerman L. "A second look at twin studies." American Psychological Association. 2004;35(4):46–47.

13. There are many differences of opinion in the "genetics versus environment" debate on the inheritance of complex characters. I had many conversation on this topic with Luca Cavalli-Sforza, the director of the Istituto di Genetica, in Pavia, Italy, where I did a post doc years ago. Cavalli-

Sforza (who many rated as the number one human geneticist in the world), argued that the twin study method was just about useless, and really told us nothing human intelligence or its control. Other researchers have reached totally opposite conclusions. Hopefully the new understanding of the epigenome will resolve this issue. Such debates in science are usually resolved not by one side or the other winning the argument, but by one side outliving the other. Cavalli-Sforza, L. *Genes, Peoples, and Languages,* trans. Mark Seielstad (New York: North Point Press; 2000). Johnson W, Turkheimer E, Gottesman II, Bouchard TJ Jr. "Beyond heritability: twin studies in behavioral research." *Curr Dir Psychol Sci.* 2010;18(4):217–20.

14. Jiang YH, et al. "Detection of clinically relevant genetic variants in autism spectrum disorder by whole-genome sequencing." *Am J Hum Genet.* 2013;93(2). These authors identified a large number of potentially important autism-related genes in whole genome sequencing of 32 families with autistic members.

15. Mameza MG, et al. "SHANK3 mutations associated with autism facilitate ligand binding to the Shank3 Ankyrin repeat region." *J Biol Chem.* 2013;288(37):26697–708.

16. See, for instance, van Wijngaarden E, et al. "Autism spectrum disorder phenotypes and prenatal exposure to methylmercury." *Epidemiology.* 2013;20(5):651–9.

17. Shelton JF, Hertz-Picciotto I, Pessah IN. "Tipping the balance of autism risk: potential mechanisms linking pesticides and autism." *Environ Health Perspect.* 2012;120 (7):944–51.

18. Landrigan PJ, Lambertini L, Birnbaum LS. "A research strategy to discover the environmental causes of autism and neurodevelopmental disabilities." *Environ Health Perspect.* 2012;120(7):a258–a260.

19. Williams E and Casanova MF. "Above genetics: lessons from cerebral development in autism." *Transl Neurosci.* 2011; 2(2):106–20.

In this review article they summarize their views of the current state of autism research, making note of the large, and unexplained increase in the incidence of autism and the need of autism researchers to understand how environmental factors affect the extremely fragile process of embryonic development of the nervous system. They further stress that if molecules occurring naturally or synthetically in our environment can affect this complex process, it may be that some of these molecules are actually necessary for the process of embryonic development to proceed unhampered.

Chapter 10

1. Ntanasis-Stathopoulos J, et al. "Epigenetic regulation on gene expression induced by physical exercise." *Musculoskelet Neuronal Interact* 2013;13(2):133–46.

2. Sanchis-Gomar F, et al. "Physical exercise as an epigenetic modulator: Eustress, the 'positive stress' as an effector of gene expression." *J Strength Cond Res* 2012;26 (12):3469–72.

3. Moore SC, et al. "Leisure time physical activity of moderate to vigorous intensity and mortality: a large pooled cohort analysis." *PLoS Med.* 2012;9(11).

4. Werner C, et al. "Physical exercise prevents cellular senescence in circulating leukocytes and in the vessel wall." *Circulation* 2009;120(24):2438–47.

5. You may wonder why this book does not include a discussion of cardiology and epigenetics. There are some papers published in this area, and it is clear that in the future it will be an important area of investigation. However, at this time there is very little solid information on the on the relationship between pathological cardiovascular states and epigenetic alterations. I spoke with several cardiologists concerning their interest in epigenetics, and they indicated that while they are aware of the field, it does not at this time have clinical implications for their activities. Leach IM, et al. "Pharmacoepigenetics in heart failure." *Curr Heart Fail Rep.* 2010;7(2):83–90.

6. Ellison GM, Waring CD, Vicinanza C, Torella D. "Physiological cardiac remod-

elling in response to endurance exercise training: cellular and molecular mechanisms." *Heart.* 2012;98(1):5–10.

7. Rönn T, et al. "A six months exercise intervention influences the genome-wide DNA methylation pattern in human adipose tissue." *PLoS Genet.* 2013;9(6).

Chapter 11

1. And it appears that most of our knowledge concerning the relationship between aging and epigenetics has been acquired in the last 15 years. There were about 200 peer reviewed publications on epigenetics and aging listed on PubMed in 2012, and just 9 published in 1998. Of course this search may have missed some articles, but these numbers certainly speak to the vast explosion scientific information that has occurred in the last few years.

2. All these figures come from Wikipedia, but there are many sources, and the numbers agree closely. There is general agreement that older lobsters are more fertile than younger lobsters, and they retain their telomeres. They add muscle throughout life as they shed their exoskeletons and increase in size. It is difficult (and risky) to determine the age of a lobster, but some lobster afficionados claim that large ones may be at least 50 years old. Lobsters as large as 22 kg have been recorded. See http://www.huffingtonpost.com/2012/11/30/lobster-age_n_2215990.html for additional details.

3. "Jeanne Calment, World's Elder, Dies at 122." Accessed August 28, 2013, http://www.nytimes.com/1997/08/05/world/jeanne-calment-world-s-elder-dies-at-122.html.

4. McKinlay, JB, McKinlay SM. "The Questionable Contribution of Medical Measures to the Decline of Mortality in the United States in the Twentieth Century." *The Milbank Memorial Fund Quarterly. Health and Society.* 1997;55(3):405–428. http://www.jstor.org/discover/10.2307/3349539?uid=3739680&uid=2&uid=4&uid=3739256&sid=21102109130433. This is a classic paper demonstrating

that most of the decline in mortality in the 20th century occurred years before the medical advances for treating specific diseases, such as vaccination and antibiotics. But now, most of the public health improvements have been made (in the industrialized countries, at least), so the question is, are the trillions of dollars we spend on health technology destined to bring about marked changes in longevity? This is, of course, one of the questions raised by this book.

5. Medvedev, Z. A. "An attempt at a rational classification of theories of aging." *Biol. Rev.* 1990;65(375):375–98.

I had the good fortune to meet Zhores Medvedev on a trip to the National Research Council Mill Hill research facility outside of London in 1982. He is well known for his analysis of the aging process and was at the forefront of development of aging theories during this period. He had had a tumultuous life as a biologist and dissident in the Soviet Union. His father was an academician who was arrested during Stalinist times and died in the gulag. He wrote many whistle blower books and articles during this period, for which he was persecuted by the Soviet government and eventually forced to move to England. He was stripped of his Russian citizenship, but it was reinstated by Gorbachev in the 1990s.

We enjoyed a wide-ranging discussion on science and politics. I was amazed that he had been able to do science that was competitive on an international level in the face of implacable treatment by the Soviet authorities.

6. Weismann also carried out critical experiments disproving the inheritance of acquired characteristics (see Chapter 1). He cut off the tails of mice (the acquired character) and noted that the offspring were always born with tails, no matter how many generations he carried on the process. While rather simplistic by today's standards, these observations were pivotal in establishing the foundation of modern genetics. Of course we see now with the rise of epigenetics that the question is much more nuanced and complex.

7. Mitteldorf J. "Aging is not a process of wear and tear." *Rejuvenation Research.* 2010;13(2–3):322–6.

8. Stocum DL and Cameron JA. "Looking proximally and distally: 100 years of limb regeneration and beyond." *Dev Dyn.* 2011;240(5):943–68. Regeneration in salamanders has been studied for the last 100 years. When a limb is amputated, the animal organizes an area called a blastema at the site that receives chemical signals and proceeds to direct the growth of a replacement limb. This obviously does not occur in most multicellular creatures, although its duplication in humans is the ambitious goal of scientists who study this process. It is difficult to understand why an ability with so much obvious survival advantage is not universal among the animal kingdom.

9. Hütter E, et al. "Oxidative stress and mitochondrial impairment can be separated from lipofuscin accumulation in aged human skeletal muscle." *Aging Cell.* 2007; 6(2):245–56.

10. Another early proposal of a somatic mutation theory of aging was put forth by Leo Szilard, "On the nature of the aging process." *Proc Natl Acad Sci U S A.* 1959; 45:30–45. Szilard was a Hungarian-American physicist who was one of the primary developers of the theory of the nuclear chain reaction responsible for the power of atomic weapons. Szilard and Robert Oppenheimer convinced Einstein to write the historic letter to President Roosevelt, encouraging him to pursue the development of the atomic bomb. After the war, Szilard and many other scientists who worked on the Manhattan Project had profound misgivings about their role in the development of such a destructive device. Szilard founded the Council for a Livable World, a lobbying group that continues today to support senate candidates who press for arms control legislation. The Council was perhaps the most committed supporter of Senator Richard Lugar of Indiana, renowned for many years as the Senate's foremost authority on arms control. Lugar was defeated in the 2012 primary by Richard Mourdock, a Tea Party candidate who went on to lose the general election to Democrat Joe Donnelly.

11. Shay JW, Wright WE. "Hayflick, his limit, and cellular aging." *Nat Rev Mol Cell Biol.* 1(2000):72–6.

12. Wright WE, Shay JW. "Telomere dynamics in cancer progression and prevention: Fundamental differences in human and mouse telomere biology." *Nature Med.* 2000;6(8): 849–851.

13. Rae MJ, et al. "The demographic and biomedical case for late-life interventions in aging." *Sci Transl Med.* 2010;2 (40):40cm21. As you can imagine, there is a booming market of anti-aging products. Some of these, such as human growth hormone, are untested in aging humans and may be potentially dangerous. It would take another book of this length to thoroughly review this controversy, but at this time there is no authenticated therapy that has yet been proven to slow, stop or reverse human aging.

14. Muller HJ. "The remaking of chromosomes." *The Collecting Net-Woods Hole.* 13(1938): 181–98.

15. Sinclair DA, Oberdoerffer P. "The ageing epigenome: damaged beyond repair?" *Ageing Res Rev.* 2009;8(3):189–98.

16. Armanios M. "Syndromes of telomere shortening." *Annu Rev Genomics Hum. Genet.* 2009;10: 45–61.

17. Carnes BA, Olshansky SJ, Hayflick L. "Can human biology allow most of us to become centenarians?" *Gerontol A Biol Sci Med Sci.* 2013;68(2):136–42 and Hayflick L. "Biological aging is no longer an unsolved problem." *Ann N Y Acad Sci.* 2007;1100:1–13. This concept combines elements of the "wear and tear" theory with the "somatic mutation" theory.

18. Lapasset L., et al. "Rejuvenating senescent and centenarian human cells by reprogramming through the pluripotent state." *Genes Dev.* 2011;25(21):2248–53. LeMaitre's exact statement was: while "Hayflick demonstrated the concept of replicative senescence, it is now clear that before this senescence-caused growth arrest, the cells age and accumulate epige-

netic changes that dramatically influence their gene expression profile leading to a 'signature of cellular aging.' But as we showed, this is clearly reprogrammable because it is based primarily on chromatin reorganization. It also means that accumulation of somatic mutations cannot explain cellular or tissue aging. We have repeated these experiments on numerous occasions. We are trying to understand further the mechanism involved, but our most important goal at present is to reconstruct a fully rejuvenated tissue and also to rejuvenate a senescent tissue."

19. I serve on the Institutional Biosafety Committee at Cincinnati Children's Hospital, which has a very large program of research in basic and medical science. IBC committees are established all over the U.S. and serve as review boards for proposed experiments involving the use of recombinant DNA funded through the federal government. Their purpose is to ensure that the research does not pose undue hazards to patients, workers or the environment. Gene transfer protocols are so widespread these days that virtually every protocol we review involves the use of viral vectors for moving genes into cells.

20. S. Jay Olshansky, Leonard Hayflick, and Bruce A. Carnes, three prominent aging researchers, stated the following in their position paper: "Our language on this matter must be unambiguous: there are no lifestyle changes, surgical procedures, vitamins, antioxidants, hormones or techniques of genetic engineering available today that have been demonstrated to influence the processes of human aging. We strongly urge the general public to avoid buying or using products or other interventions from anyone claiming that they will slow, stop or reverse aging." Olshansky SJ, Hayflick L, Carnes BA. "Position statement on human aging." *J Gerontol A Biol Sci Med Sci.* 2002;57(8):B292–7.

Chapter 12

1. Shelton JF, Hertz-Picciotto I, Pessah IN. "Tipping the balance of autism risk: po-

tential mechanisms linking pesticides and autism." *Environ Health Perspect.* 2012;120 (7):944–51.

2. The American Chemical Council, an industry lobbying group, has carried on an active campaign over the years to fight legislation restricting the use of BPA.

3. Schlager G, Dickie MM. "Spontaneous mutations and mutation rates in the house mouse." *Genetics.* 196757(2):319–30. Over the years there has been a mountain of research on the health effects of coffee and caffeine. Despite all this effort there is at present no consensus on the health effects of coffee; some studies suggest some cardiovascular risk, yet other research failed to support such conclusions. Many of the early studies were flawed due to the fact that at the time they were carried out, most coffee drinkers were also cigarette smokers, and this contribution was not properly factored out. Despite the fact that it is perhaps the most effective and widely used stimulant known to humanity, its long term health effects appear to be modest to non-existent. See Chou T. "Wake up and smell the coffee: Caffeine, coffee, and the medical consequences." *West J Med.* 1992;157(5):544–53. Extensive trials have never shown caffeine to be a mutagen in mammals (Timson J. "Caffeine." *Mutat Res.* 1997;47(1):1–52). This is indeed surprising, as it inhibits the DNA repair process in bacteria.

4. Ames BN, Lee FD, Durston WE. "An improved bacterial test system for the detection and classification of mutagens and carcinogens." *Proc Natl Acad Sci U S A.* 1973;70(73):782–6.

5. McCann J, Ames BN. "Detection of carcinogens as mutagens in the Salmonella/microsome test: assay of 300 chemicals: discussion." *Proc Natl Acad Sci U S A.* 1976;73(3):950–4.

6. Hengstler JG, et al. "Critical evaluation of key evidence on the human health hazards of exposure to bisphenol A." *Crit Rev Toxicol.* 2011;41(4):263–91. This paper is an extensive review article concluding that BPA levels in the environment pose no hazard. However, there are many studies

that argue to the contrary. See Bernal AJ, Jirtle RL. "Epigenomic disruption: the effects of early developmental exposures." *Birth Defects Res A Clin Mol Teratol.* 2010;88(10):938–44.

7. Vandenberg LN, et al. "Urinary, circulating, and tissue biomonitoring studies indicate widespread exposure to bisphenol A." *Cien Saude Colet.* 2012;17(2):407–34. The authors reach much the same conclusion that I will present in the concluding chapters: there is substantial controversy, gaps in our knowledge and a crying need for more research.

8. There are a large number of conservative think tanks that produce position papers and research conclusively proving that environmental regulations are onerous, too expensive, obstruct capitalism and are unnecessary, because there is nothing in the environment that can be a significant factor in cancer or mutation causation. Check out. for example, http://www.cato.org/publications/commentary/congress-needs-realize-environment-doesnt-cause-cancer for some out of date information on this topic.

9. Mishra S, Dwivedi AR, Prakash S, Singh RB. "Review on Epigenetic Effect of Heavy Metal Carcinogens on Human Health." *Open Nutraceuticals Journal.* 2010 (3):188.

10. Hormones can also be large protein molecules, such as insulin and human growth hormone, but that's another story, and we won't delve into it here.

11. See "TEDX List of Potential Endocrine Disruptors," accessed August 29, 2013, http://www.endocrinedisruption.com/endocrine.TEDXList.overview.php for a list of 870 such substances.

12. LeBlanc GA. "Are environmental sentinels signaling?" *Environ Health Perspect.* 1995;103(10):888–90.

13. Flint S, Markle T, Thompson S, Wallace E. "Bisphenol A exposure, effects, and policy: a wildlife perspective." *J Environ Manage.* 2012;15(104):19–34.

14. Patisaul HB, Adewale HB. "Long-term effects of environmental endocrine disruptors on reproductive physiology and behavior." *Front Behav Neurosci.* 2009; 3:10.

15. Davis WP, Bortone SA. "Effects of kraft mill effluent on the sexuality of fishes: an environmental early warning?" *Chemically-Induced Alterations in Sexual and Functional Development: The Wildlife/Human Connection.* Eds. Colborn T, Clements C (Princeton: Princeton Scientific; 1972), 113–127.

16. Readers are probably aware of the controversy over insecticides, of which DDT was the 1960s poster child of environmental demolition derbies. The push against insecticides such as DDT was driven in large part by Rachel Carson's famous book, *Silent Spring*, voicing concerns over the widespread use of these agents. Carson never advocated banning DDT, a point missed by her present day critics, but she did caution against its overuse. The big shortcoming of such agents is that they are very stable and long-lived, and build up in the food chain. In the case of bird populations at the top of the food chain (raptors, including falcons and other birds of prey) this resulted in high concentrations of DDT accumulating in the birds' tissues, interfering with their ability to form their eggshells. DDT and related compounds are endocrine disruptors and interfere with normal female reproductive function. In addition to their destructive effects on bird populations, these compounds destroy virtually all insects, 99 percent or more of which are not harmful, and in some cases highly beneficial.

Another misconception is that Carson's book alone was responsible for the banning of DDT in the United States (it was never banned in Africa and is still manufactured in the US). During the 60s there were thousands of scientific papers published on the topic, there were congressional hearings, thousands of hours of testimony, and a massive public reaction against the misuse of chemicals for controlling insects. After DDT was banned in the 1960s the catastrophic decline of raptor populations ceased, and despite many threats to their survival, healthy number have been reestablished. Although concern over loss of bird species motivated public support for a ban of DDT, the real reason for its declining use has been its ineffectiveness due to the emergence of insect populations resistant to DDT and related pesticides.

17. Just how politically tangled these issues have become is shown by the recent flap over birth control pills as the cause of disruption of reproductive function in fish. Anti-birth control websites have circulated stories stating that decline in fish populations is due to environmental contamination from the urine of women using birth control pills. However, there is no sound science to back up this claim, and the level of endocrine disruptor compounds released into the environment from agricultural and industrial sources is thousands of times greater than that contributed by users of birth control devices.

This debate has been going on for several years and reinforces my central message: we need sound science to establish these links, we need to look at remediation that is successful and cost effective, and the burden of the cost must be shouldered by those who are causing the problem.

For a thoughtful and balanced analysis of the issue see Moore K, McGuire KI, Gordon R, Woodruff TJ. "Birth control hormones in water: separating myth from fact." *Contraception*, 2011;84(2):115–8.

18. "US Fish and Wildlife Service Environmental Quality: Endocrine Disruptors." Accessed August 29, 2013. http://www.fws.gov/contaminants/issues/EndocrineDisruptors.cfm.

19. McLachlan JA. "Environmental signaling: what embryos and evolution teach us about endocrine disrupting chemicals." *Endocr Rev.* 2001;22(3):319–41.

20. Bollati V, Baccarelli A. "Environmental epigenetics." *Heredity (Edinb).* 2010;105(1):105–12.

21. Manikkam M, Tracey R, Guerrero-Bosagna C, Skinner MK. "Plastics derived endocrine disruptors (BPA, DEHP and DBP) induce epigenetic transgenerational inheritance of obesity, reproductive disease and sperm epimutations." *PLoS One.* 2013; 8(1).

Chapter 13

1. "Bill McKibben, Global Warming's Terrifying New Math." Accessed August 30, 2013. http://www.rollingstone.com/politics/news/global-warmings-terrifying-new-math-20120719.

2. "CNN Opinion: A meteor and asteroid: 1 in 100 million odds." Accessed August 30, 2013. http://www.cnn.com/2013/02/16/opinion/urry-meteor-asteroid.

3. "WWF: How many species are we losing?" Accessed Aug 30, 2013, http://wwf.panda.org/about_our_earth/biodiversity/biodiversity/.

4. "The Falling-Bridge Lesson: The U.S. Infrastructure Failure Is Still Totally Inexcusable." Accessed August 30, 2013. http://www.theatlantic.com/business/archive/2013/05/the-falling-bridge-lesson-the-us-infrastructure-failure-is-still-totally-inexcusable/276220/.

5. The U.N. Food and Agriculture's Report on the state of the world's aquaculture concludes that about 50 percent of all marine fish stocks are being "fully exploited"—meaning they are being fished at or near sustainable limits. Another 19 percent are overexploited, eight percent depleted and one percent recovering from depletion. Other reports predict the collapse of the ocean ecosystem because of overfishing of the smallest fish in the ocean that reside at the bottom of the food chain. "Overfishing: a threat to marine biodiversity." Accessed August 30, 2013. http://www.un.org/events/tenstories/06/story.asp?storyID=800.

6. Politifact and many other fact checking organizations list laudatory praise of U.S. healthcare by numerous American politicians. Over and over again the U.S. falls way down on the list, depending on the criteria employed. There is no nonpartisan, objective assessment that puts the U.S. healthcare system at the top. "John Boehner says U.S. health care system is best in world." Accessed August 30, 2013. http://

www.politifact.com/truth-o-meter/
statements/2012/jul/05/john-boehner/john-
boehner-says-us-health-care-system-best-
world/.

7. "Health at a glance: Europe 2012."
Accessed August 30, 2013. http://www.
oecd.org/els/health-systems/HealthAtA
GlanceEurope2012.pdf.

8. Haig D. "Weismann Rules! OK? Epigenetics and the Lamarckian temptation."
Biology and Philosophy. 2007; 22:415–28.

9. Over the years the term "gay gene"
had scooted into the public consciousness,
the idea that a single mutant gene could determine sexual orientation. This is the
dumbest, most naïve reading of genetics
ever promulgated on the public. It is absolutely impossible that a pattern of behavior so complex, and so dependent on environmental influences could be determined
by "a" gene.

10. Remember that we are talking about
the range of variation in IQ throughout the
population as a whole. If you looked at a distribution of IQ scores, you would see a bell-
shaped curve, with 100 as the most frequent
value. There are of course mutations that
cause very serious mental retardation, and
in most cases they are well understood at
the molecular level. Their values are off the
lower left hand end of the scale, and they
may result from biochemical disorders,
in which an enzyme is absent or nonfunctional as in the case of phenylke-
tonuria. The problem with trying to study
the normal range of variation is that each
gene makes only a tiny contribution to IQ
values, and many studies aimed at identifying genes for IQ have proved difficult to
replicate.

11. Yu CC, et al. "Genome-wide DNA
methylation and gene expression analyses
of monozygotic twins discordant for intelligence levels." *PLoS One.* 2012;7(10).

12. Greiffenstein MF. "Secular IQ increases by epigenesis? The hypothesis of
cognitive genotype optimization." *Psychol
Rep.* 2011;109(2):353–66. The author proposes that overall increases in the IQ of the
population may be driven by epigenetic
feedback as I suggested.

13. Sometimes families struggling with
a catastrophic disease affecting their child
may take steps that are so heroic that they
become scenarios for Hollywood films.
Several years ago I wrote an article for *Biopharm International* (volume 24, Issue 5, p.
50) describing two films that take on this
difficult topic, both "based on true events"
(http://www.biopharminternational.com/
biopharm/article/articleDetail.jsp?id=
718074).

The films have many similarities. *Lorenzo's
Oil* (Universal Pictures; Directed by George
Miller) and *Extraordinary Measures* (CBS
Films; Directed by Tom Vaughn) both de-
pict families who attempt to discover and
implement cures for their children's genetic
diseases when they find no remedy in current medical science. Both are beautifully
filmed and edited. Both present a great
amount of scientific detail and make a
powerful case for the lavish support that
medical research enjoys. Both have feel-
good endings that, amazingly enough, turn
out to be largely accurate. One of the most
interesting aspects of the two films, when
compared with one another, was how much
the science had changed, between 1992
(when *Lorenzo's Oil* was made) and 2010,
which saw the release of *Extraordinary
Measures.*

14. "Obama seeking to boost study of
the human brain." Accessed August 30,
2013. http://www.nytimes.com/2013/02/18/
science/project-seeks-to-build-map-of-
human-brain.html?pagewanted=all&_r=0.

15. "Michael J. Fox Foundation Parkinson's funded grant: DNA Methylation as an
Epigenetic Mechanism in the Etiopatho-
genesis of Parkinson's Disease." Accessed
August 30, 2013, https://www.michaeljfox.
org/foundation/grant-detail.php?grant_id=
400.

16. Healy A, Rush R, Ocain T. "Fragile
X syndrome: an update on developing
treatment modalities." *ACS Chem Neurosci.*
2011;2(8):402–10.

17. Their website (http://sfari.org/fund
ing/grants) states: "We solicit applications
for SFARI Awards from individuals who will
conduct bold, imaginative, rigorous and rel-

evant research in three main research areas: cognition and behavior, gene discovery and molecular mechanisms." I couldn't have said it better myself. "Simons Foundation Autism Research Initiative: Funding." http://sfari.org/news-and-opinion/news/2013/twin-study-finds-epigenetic-imprint-of-autism-traits).

18. According to the CDC, cigarette smoking is the number one (but not the only) risk factor for lung cancer, responsible for 90 percent of cases. Smokers are 15 to 30 times more likely to get lung cancer or die from lung cancer than people who do not smoke. Every year in the United States, about 3,000 people who never smoked die from lung cancer due to secondhand smoke. Radon is a naturally occurring gas that comes from rocks and dirt and may accumulate in houses and buildings. Radon causes about 20,000 cases of lung cancer each year, making it the second leading cause of lung cancer. Nearly one out of every 15 homes in the U.S. is estimated to have high radon levels. "CDC: Lung cancer risk factors." Accessed August 30, 2013. http://www.cdc.gov/cancer/lung/basic_info/risk_factors.htm.

19. Ntanasis-Stathopoulos J, et al. "Epigenetic regulation on gene expression induced by physical exercise." *J Musculoskelet Neuronal Interact.* 2012;13(2):133–46.

20. Cummings KM, Brown A, O'Connor R. "The cigarette controversy." *Cancer Epidemiol Biomarkers Prev.* 2007;16:1070–6.

Chapter 14

1. I have emphasized my belief throughout this book that our government needs to do more, but the reader should not think from this complaint that I believe the government is doing nothing. A recent review of genomics and epigenomics discusses the ENCODE project, a very large scale analysis of data from both genomic and epigenomic sources. The author explains that "the data from epigenome studies are providing information of far greater significance than simply mapping specific epigenetic marks to a given cell type. Key

applications are related to genome annotation, cell identity and disease. The project demonstrates that investigations based on the primary DNA sequence alone cannot provide a comprehensive understanding of the mammalian genome. Chromatin signatures (see Chapter 1), for example, allow precise genome annotation of regulatory elements and locate functional or cell type-specific regions of interest. Precise chromatin states can clarify a gene's activity status, which in turn has consequences for how specific gene loci behave in normal development and disease. See Dauncey MJ. "Genomic and Epigenomic Insights into Nutrition and Brain Disorders." *Nutrients.* 2013;5:887–914.

Another megascience project that embraces epigenetics is the *NIH Roadmap Epigenomics Program* (http://www.roadmapepigenomics.org), which is conducting in-depth epigenomic mapping of several high-priority human cell types. The work will investigate over 30 histone modifications using state-of-the-art sequencing technology. Some of these findings on human cell lines grown in culture have already been published.

2. "The Texas Tribune, Texas Scientists Regret Loss of Higgs Boson Quest." Accessed August 30, 2013. http://www.texastribune.org/texas-taxes/budget/higgs-boson-discovery-may-have-been-possible-texas/.

3. According to Batelle, China is on track to overtake the U.S. in R&D spending by 2020. http://www.computerworld.com/s/article/9234976/China_set_to_surpass_U.S._in_R_D_spending_in_10_years_.

4. In discussions with administrators at NIH, they have indicated to me that they have cut back on major programs in an effort to save the individual investigator grants. This may work as a stopgap measure, but everyone recognizes that if the NIH budget is cut year after year eventually there will be nothing left to cut.

5. "NASA: Mars exploration program." Accessed August 30, 2013. http://mars.jpl.nasa.gov/news/whatsnew/. The website describes in detail the design of the spacecraft

and includes videos showing the final minutes of its landing maneuvers. The engineering challenges are incredible.

Chapter 15

1. Greally JM and Jacobs MN. "State of the Science on in vitro and in vivo testing methods of epigenomic endpoints for evaluating endocrine disruptors."*ALTEX*, published online. June 20, 2013. S18686 96X1302211X.This is an extensive and detailed paper in which the authors discuss a number of options for screening for epimutagenic chemicals.

2. As of the end of 2013 there are 31,857 references in the Medline search listed under the heading of "epigenetic."

3. The term "cure" is bandied about frequently when news reports of cancer treatments appear. A cure would mean a complete removal of the cancer. A "cure" is extremely unlikely, for reasons discussed in this book. Cancer specialists look for therapies that will slow or hold back malignancies. Currently it is generally accepted that the best that can be hoped for in the short run is a truce with cancer, similar to the AIDS/HIV situation.

Selected Bibliography

Ally D, Ritland K, Otto SP. "Aging in a long-lived clonal tree." *PLoS Biol.* 2010; 8(8):782–6.

Ames BN, Lee FD, Durston WE. "An improved bacterial test system for the detection and classification of mutagens and carcinogens." *Proc Natl Acad Sci U S A.* 1973;70(73):782–6.

Armanios M. "Syndromes of telomere shortening." *Annu Rev Genomics Hum. Genet.* 2009;10: 45–61.

Bakulski KM, et al. "*Genome-wide DNA methylation differences between late-onset Alzheimer's disease and cognitively normal controls in human frontal cortex.*" *J Alzheimers Dis.* 2012;29(3): 571–88.

Bakulski KM, Rozek LS, Dolinoy DC, Paulson HL, Hu H. "*Alzheimer's disease and environmental exposure to lead: The epidemiologic evidence and potential role of epigenetics.*" *Curr Alzheimer Res.* 2012;9(5):563–73.

Bird SC. "Towards improvements in the estimation of the coalescent: implications for the most effective use of Y chromosome short tandem repeat mutation rates." *PLoS One.* 2012;7 (10).

Blumenthal T. "Operons in eukaryotes." *Brief Funct Genomic Proteomic.* (2004)3(3):199–211.

Bollati V, Baccarelli A. "Environmental epigenetics." *Heredity (Edinb).* 2010; 105(1):105–12.

Bota, S., et al. "Follow-up of bronchial precancerous lesions and carcinoma *in situ* using fluorescence endoscopy." *Am J Respir Crit Care Med.* 2001;164 (9):1688–93.

Brenner DJ, Hall EJ. "Computed tomography—an increasing source of radiation exposure." *N Engl J Med.* 2007; 357(22):2277–84.

Brewer GJ. "The risks of copper toxicity contributing to cognitive decline in the aging population and to Alzheimer's disease." *J Am Coll Nutr.* 2009;28(3): 238–42.

Briggs R, King TJ. "Nuclear transplantation studies on the early gastrula (Rana pipiens) I. Nuclei of presumptive endoderm." *Dev Biol.* 1960;2(3): 252–70.

Buxhoeveden DP, Casanova MF. "The minicolumn hypothesis in neuroscience." *Brain.* 2002;125(Pt 5):935–51.

Carlson EA. "H.J. Muller's contributions to mutation research." *Mutat Res.* 2013. 752(1):1–5.

Carlsson HE, Schapiro SJ, Farah I, Hau J. "Use of primates in research: a global overview." *Am J Primatol.* 2004;63(4): 225–37.

Carnes BA, Olshansky SJ, Hayflick L. "Can human biology allow most of us to become centenarians?" *Gerontol A Biol Sci Med Sci.* 2013;68(2):136–42.

Cavalli-Sforza, L. *Genes, Peoples, and Languages.* Trans. Mark Seielstad. New York: North Point Press; 2000.

Chou T. "Wake up and smell the coffee: Caffeine, coffee, and the medical consequences." *West J Med.* 1992;157(5): 544–53.

Copeland RA, Moyer MP, Richon VM.

"Targeting genetic alterations in protein methyltransferases for personalized cancer therapeutics." *Oncogene.* 2013;32(8):939–46.

Corcellis J, et al. "The aftermath of boxing." *Psychol Med.* 1973;3(3):270–303.

Cribbs DH. "Abeta DNA vaccination for Alzheimer's disease: focus on disease prevention." *CNS Neurol Disord Drug Targets.* 2010;9(2):207–16.

Cummings KM, Brown A, O'Connor R. "The cigarette controversy." *Cancer Epidemiol Biomarkers Prev.* 2007;16: 1070–6.

Daubriac JD, et al. "Molecular changes in mesothelioma with an impact on prognosis and treatment." *Arch Pathol Lab Med.* 2012;136(3):277–93.

Dauncey MJ. "Genomic and Epigenomic Insights into Nutrition and Brain Disorders." *Nutrients.* 2013;5:887–914.

Davis WP, Bortone SA., "Effects of kraft mill effluent on the sexuality of fishes: an environmental early warning?" 1992. In: *Chemically-Induced Alterations in Sexual and Functional Development: The Wildlife/Human Connection.* Edited by Colborn T, Clements C (Princeton Scientific Publishing Co, Inc, Princeton, NJ, pp 113–127.

Dolinoy DC, Huang D, Jirtle RL. "Maternal nutrient supplementation counteracts bisphenol A-induced DNA hypomethylation in early development." *Proc Natl Acad Sci U S A.* 2007;104(42):13056–61.

Dyer C. "Flu vaccine investigator is suspended for four months for research fraud." *BMJ.* 2012;16.

Ellison GM, Waring CD, Vicinanza C, Torella D. "Physiological cardiac remodelling in response to endurance exercise training: cellular and molecular mechanisms." *Heart.* 2012;98(1):5–10.

Faras H, Al Ateeqi N, Tidmarsh L. "Autism spectrum disorders." *Ann Saudi Med.* 2010;30(4):295–300.

Ferreira PC, Piai Kde A, Takayanagui AM, Segura-Muñoz SI. "Aluminum as a risk factor for Alzheimer's disease." *Rev Lat Am Enfermagem.* 2008;16(1): 151–7.

Flint S, Markle T, Thompson S, Wallace E. "Bisphenol A exposure, effects, and policy: a wildlife perspective." *J Environ Manage.* 2012;15(104):19–34.

Forsberg PA, Mark TM. "Pomalidomide in the treatment of relapsed multiple myeloma." *Future Oncol.* 2013;9(7): 939–48.

Frances A. *Saving Normal: An Insider's Revolt Against Out-of-Control Psychiatric Diagnosis, DSM-5, Big Pharma, and the Medicalization of Ordinary Life.* New York: William Morrow; 2013.

Golde TE, et al. "Alzheimer's disease risk alleles in TREM2 illuminate innate immunity in Alzheimer's disease." *Alzheimers Res Ther.* 2013;5(3):24.

Gos M. "Epigenetic mechanisms of gene expression regulation in neurological diseases." *Acta Neurobiol Exp (Wars).* 2013;73(1):19–37.

Gräff J, et al. "An epigenetic blockade of cognitive functions in the neurodegenerating brain." *Nature.* 2012; 483 (7388):222–6.

Greiffenstein MF. "Secular IQ increases by epigenesis? The hypothesis of cognitive genotype optimization." *Psychol Rep.* 2011;109(2):353–66.

Gu Y, Scarmeas N. "Dietary patterns in Alzheimer's disease and cognitive aging." *Curr Alzheimer Res.* 2011;8(5): 510–9.

Gurdon JB. "The cloning of a frog." *Development.* 2013;140(12):2446–8.

Haig D. "Weismann Rules! OK? Epigenetics and the Lamarckian temptation." *Biology and Philosophy.* 2007; 22:415–28.

Harith HH, Morris MJ, Kavurma MM. "On the TRAIL of obesity and diabetes." *Trends Endocrinol Metab.* 2013; 24(11):578–87.

Hayflick L. "Biological aging is no longer an unsolved problem." *Ann N Y Acad Sci.* 2007;1100:1–13.

Healy A, Rush R, Ocain T. "Fragile × syndrome: an update on developing treatment modalities." *ACS Chem Neurosci.* 2011;2(8):402–10.

Hengstler JG, et al. "Critical evaluation of key evidence on the human health hazards of exposure to bisphenol A." *Crit Rev Toxicol.* 2011;41(4):263–91.

Hoek HW, et al. "Schizoid personality disorder after prenatal exposure to famine." *Am J Psychiatry.* 1996;153(12): 1637–39.

Hoppe PC, Illmensee K. "Full-term development after transplantation of parthenogenetic embryonic nuclei into fertilized mouse eggs." *Proc Natl Acad Sci U S A.* 1982;79(6):1912–6.

Hütter E, et al. "Oxidative stress and mitochondrial impairment can be separated from lipofuscin accumulation in aged human skeletal muscle." *Aging Cell.* 2007;6(2):245–56.

Insel TR, Wang PS. "The STAR*D trial: revealing the need for better treatments." *Psychiatr Serv.* 2009;60(11): 1466–7.

Jiang YH, et al. "Detection of clinically relevant genetic variants in autism spectrum disorder by whole-genome sequencing." *Am J Hum Genet.* 2013;93 (2).

Johnson W, Turkheimer E, Gottesman II, Bouchard TJ Jr. "Beyond heritability: twin studies in behavioral research." *Curr Dir Psychol Sci.* 2010;18 (4):217–20.

Karagiannis TC and Ververis K. "Potential of chromatin modifying compounds for the treatment of Alzheimer's disease." *Pathobiol Aging Age Relat Dis.* 2012;2(10).

Kevles, DJ. *In the Name of Eugenics: Genetics and the Uses of Human Heredity.* Cambridge: Harvard University Press; 1998.

Kim K, Park H. "Association between urinary concentrations of bisphenol A and type 2 diabetes in Korean adults: a population-based cross-sectional study." *Int J Hyg Environ Health.* 2013;216(4):467–71.

Kim S., et al. "The preventive and therapeutic effects of intravenous human adipose-derived stem cells in Alzheimer's disease mice." *PLoS One.* 2012;7(9):1–17.

Kirkbride JB, et al. "Prenatal nutrition, epigenetics and schizophrenia risk: can we test causal effects?" *Epigenomics.* 2012;4(3):303–15.

Konsoula Z, Barile FA. "Epigenetic histone acetylation and deacetylation mechanisms in experimental models of neurodegenerative disorders." *J Pharmacol Toxicol Methods.* 2012;66(3):215–20.

Kuhn T. *The Structure of Scientific Revolutions.* Chicago: University of Chicago Press; 1962.

Kurttio P, et al. "Fallout from the Chernobyl accident and overall cancer incidence in Finland." *Cancer Epidemiol.* 2013;7(5):585–92.

Lahav R. "Endothelin receptor B is required for the expansion of melanocyte precursors and malignant melanoma." *Int J Dev Biol.* 2005;49(2–3):173–80.

Landrigan PJ, Lambertini L, Birnbaum LS. "A research strategy to discover the environmental causes of autism and neurodevelopmental disabilities." *Environ Health Perspect.* 2012;120(7): a258–a260.

Lapasset L., et al. "Rejuvenating senescent and centenarian human cells by reprogramming through the pluripotent state." *Genes Dev.* 2011;25(21): 2248–53.

Latini G, Ferri M, Chiellini F. "Materials degradation in PVC medical devices, DEHP leaching and neonatal outcomes." *Curr Med Chem.* 2010;17(26): 2979–89.

Leach IM, et al. "Pharmacoepigenetics in heart failure." *Curr Heart Fail Rep.* 2010;7(2):83–90.

LeBlanc GA. "Are environmental sentinels signaling?" *Environ Health Perspect.* 1995;103(10):888–90.

Lewis DA, Sweet RA. "Schizophrenia from a neural circuitry perspective: advancing toward rational pharmacological therapies." *J Clin Invest.* 2009; 119(4):706–16.

Ling C, Groop L. "Epigenetics: a molecular link between environmental factors and type 2 diabetes." *Diabetes.* 2009;58(12):2718–25.

Mameza MG, et al. "SHANK3 mutations associated with autism facilitate ligand binding to the Shank3 Ankyrin repeat region." *J Biol Chem.* 2013;288(37): 26697–708.

Manikkam M, Tracey R, Guerrero-Bosagna C, Skinner MK. "Plastics derived endocrine disruptors (BPA, DEHP and DBP) induce epigenetic transgenerational inheritance of obesity, reproductive disease and sperm epimutations." *PLoS One.* 2013;8(1).

McCann J, Ames BN. "Detection of carcinogens as mutagens in the Salmonella/microsome test: assay of 300 chemicals: discussion." *Proc Natl Acad Sci U S A.* 1976;73(3):950–4.

McCarrey JR. "The epigenome as a target for heritable environmental disruptions of cellular function." *Mol Cell Endocrin.* 2012; 354(1–2):9–15.

McKinlay, JB, McKinlay SM. "The Questionable Contribution of Medical Measures to the Decline of Mortality in the United States in the Twentieth Century." *The Milbank Memorial Fund Quarterly. Health and Society.* 1997;55(3):405–428.

McLachlan JA. "Environmental signaling: what embryos and evolution teach us about endocrine disrupting chemicals." *Endocr Rev.* 2001;22(3): 319–41.

Medvedev, Z. A. "An attempt at a rational classification of theories of aging." *Biol. Rev.* 1990;65(375):375–98.

Meymandi, A. "The science of epigenetics." *Psychiatry (Edgmont).* 2010;7(3): 40–41.

Mikaelsson MA, Miller CA. "DNA methylation: a transcriptional mechanism co-opted by the developed mammalian brain?" *Epigenetics.* 2011; 6(5):548–51.

Mishra S, Dwivedi AR, Prakash S, Singh RB. "Review on Epigenetic Effect of Heavy Metal Carcinogens on Human Health." *Open Nutraceuticals Journal.* 2010(3):188.

Mitteldorf J. "Aging is not a process of wear and tear." *Rejuvenation Research.* 2010;13(2–3):322–6.

Moore K, McGuire KI, Gordon R, Woodruff TJ. "Birth control hormones in water: separating myth from fact." *Contraception,* 2011;84(2):115–8.

Moore SC, et al. "Leisure time physical activity of moderate to vigorous intensity and mortality: a large pooled cohort analysis." *PLoS Med.* 2012;9(11).

Moss JB, et al. "Regeneration of the pancreas in adult zebrafish." *Diabetes.* 2009;58(8):1844–51.

Muller HJ. "The remaking of chromosomes." *The Collecting Net-Woods Hole.* 13(1938): 181–98.

Murphy SK, Jirtle RL. "Imprinting evolution and the price of silence." *Bioessays.* 2003;25(6):577–588.

Nedd, CA, 2nd. "When the solution is the problem: a brief history of the shoe fluoroscope." *AJR Am J Roentgenol.* 1992;158(6):1270.

Nikoshkov A, et al. "Epigenetic DNA methylation in the promoters of the Igf1 receptor and insulin receptor genes in db/db mice." *Epigenetics.* 2011;6(4):405–9.

Nitert MD, et al. "Impact of an exercise intervention on DNA methylation in skeletal muscle from first-degree relatives of patients with type 2 diabetes." *Diabetes.* 2012;61(12):3322–32.

Normile D, Vogel G, Couzin J. "Cloning. South Korean team's remaining human stem cell claim demolished." *Science.* 2006;11(5758):156–7.

Ntanasis-Stathopoulos J, et al. "Epigenetic regulation on gene expression induced by physical exercise." *J Musculoskelet Neuronal Interact*. 2012;13 (2):133–46.

Ogrodnik A, Hudon TW, Nadkarni PM, Chandawarkar RY. "Radiation exposure and breast cancer: lessons from Chernobyl." *Conn Med*. 2013;77(4): 227–34.

Olshansky SJ, Hayflick L, Carnes BA. "Position statement on human aging." *J Gerontol A Biol Sci Med Sci*. 2002; 57(8):B292–7.

Papavramidou, N, Papavramidis, T, and Demetriou, T. "Ancient Greek and Greco–Roman methods in modern surgical treatment of cancer." *Ann Surg Oncol*. 2010;17(3): 665–7.

Patisaul HB, Adewale HB. "Long-term effects of environmental endocrine disruptors on reproductive physiology and behavior." *Front Behav Neurosci*. 2009;3:10.

Peter CJ, Akbarian S. "Balancing histone methylation activities in psychiatric disorders." *Trends in Mol Med*. 2011;17(7):372–79.

"Questionable methods of cancer management: Electronic devices." *CA Cancer J Clin*. 1994;44(12):115–27.

Quiroga, PQ, Fried, I, Koch C. "Brain cells for grandmother." *Sci Am*. 2013; 308(2):31–5.

Rae MJ, et al. "The demographic and biomedical case for late-life interventions in aging." *Sci Transl Med*. 2010;2(40):40cm21.

Rao JS, Keleshian VL, Klein S, Rapoport SI. "Epigenetic modifications in frontal cortex from Alzheimer's disease and bipolar disorder patients." *Transl Psychiatry*. 2012;2.

Rönn T, et al. "A six months exercise intervention influences the genome-wide DNA methylation pattern in human adipose tissue." *PLoS Genet*. 2013;9(6).

Sage J., "The retinoblastoma tumor suppressor and stem cell biology," Genes Dev. 26(2012):1409–20.

St. Clair D, Xu M, Wang P, et al. "Rates of adult schizophrenia following prenatal exposure to the Chinese famine of 1959–1961." *JAMA* 2005;294(5):557–62.

Sanchis-Gomar F, et al. "Physical exercise as an epigenetic modulator: Eustress, the 'positive stress' as an effector of gene expression." *J Strength Cond Res* 2012;26(12):3469–72.

Sanghera DK, Blackett PR. "Type 2 diabetes genetics: Beyond GWAS." *J Diabetes Metab*. 2013;3(198).

Schlager G, Dickie MM. "Spontaneous mutations and mutation rates in the house mouse." *Genetics*. 196757(2):319–30.

Schulz L. "The Dutch hunger winter and the developmental origins of health and disease." *Proc Natl Acad Sci U S A*. 2010;107(39):16757–58.

Seow WJ, et al. "Urinary benzene biomarkers and DNA methylation in Bulgarian petrochemical workers: study findings and comparison of linear and beta regression models." *PLoS One*. 2012;7(12):e504.

Shankar A, Teppala S, Sabanayagam C. "Bisphenol A and peripheral arterial disease: results from the NHANES." *Environ Health Perspect*. 2012;120(9):1297–1300.

Shay JW, Wright WE. "Hayflick, his limit, and cellular ageing." *Nat Rev Mol Cell Biol*. 1(2000):72–6.

Shelton JF, Hertz-Picciotto I, Pessah IN. "Tipping the balance of autism risk: potential mechanisms linking pesticides and autism." *Environ Health Perspect*. 2012;120(7):944–51. http://www.ncbi.nlm.nih.gov/pubmed/22534084.

Shore ND, et al. "Building on sipuleucel-T for immunologic treatment of castration-resistant prostate cancer." *Cancer Control*. 2013;20(1):7–16.

Sinclair DA, Oberdoerffer P. "*The ageing epigenome: Damaged beyond repair?*" *Ageing Res Rev*. 2009;8(3):189–98.

Singh S, Li SS. "Epigenetic effects of

environmental chemicals bisphenol a and phthalates." *Int J Mol Sci.* 2012; 13(8):10143–53.

Spanos NP, Gottlieb J. "Ergotism and the Salem Village witch trials." *Science.* 1976;194(4274):1390–4.

Stent, G. S. *Molecular Genetics: An Introductory Narrative.* San Francisco: W.H. Freeman; 1971.

Stiller JW, Weinberger DR., "Boxing and chronic brain damage," Psychiatric Clinics of North America 8(1985): 339–56.

Stocum DL and Cameron JA. "Looking proximally and distally: 100 years of limb regeneration and beyond." *Dev Dyn.* 2011;240(5):943–68.

Strasak AM, et al. "Statistical errors in medical research—a review of common pitfalls." *Swiss Med Wkly.* 2007; 137(3–4):44–9.

Szilard, L. "On the nature of the aging process." *Proc Natl Acad Sci U S A.* 1959;45:30–45.

Thayer KA, et al. "Role of environmental chemicals in diabetes and obesity: a National Toxicology Program workshop review." *Environ Health Perspect.* 2012;120(6):779–89.

Timson J. "Caffeine." *Mutat Res.* 1997; 47(1):1–52.

Ujvari B, et al. "Evolution of a contagious cancer: epigenetic variation in Devil Facial Tumour Disease." *Proc Biol Sci.* 2013;280(1750):20121720.

Vandenberg LN, et al. "Urinary, circulating, and tissue biomonitoring studies indicate widespread exposure to bisphenol A." *Cien Saude Colet.* 2012; 17(2):407–34.

Vrachnis N, et al. "Impact of maternal diabetes on epigenetic modifications leading to diseases in the offspring." *Exp Diabetes Res.* 2012:538474.

Waddington CH. "The epigenotype: 1942." *Int J Epidemiol.* 2012;41(1):10–3.

Walker CL, Ho SM. "Developmental reprogramming of cancer susceptibility." *Nat Rev Cancer.* 2012;12(7):479–86.

Wei J, et al. "Perinatal exposure to bisphenol A at reference dose predisposes offspring to metabolic syndrome in adult rats on a high-fat diet." *Endocrinology.* 2011;152(8):3049–61.

Werner C, et al. "Physical exercise prevents cellular senescence in circulating leukocytes and in the vessel wall." *Circulation* 2009;120(24):2438–47.

Wilkinson DM, Ruxton GD. "Understanding selection for long necks in different taxa." *Biol Rev.* 2012;87(3): 616–30.

Williams E and Casanova MF. "Above genetics: lessons from cerebral development in autism." *Transl Neurosci.* 2011;2(2):106–20.

Wright WE, Shay JW. "Telomere dynamics in cancer progression and prevention: Fundamental differences in human and mouse telomere biology." *Nature Med.* 2000;6(8): 849–851.

Wurz GT, et al. "Antitumor effects of L-BLP25 Antigen-Specific tumor immunotherapy in a novel human MUC1 transgenic lung cancer mouse model." *J Transl Med.* 2013;11(1):64.

Yablokov AV. "Chernobyl's radioactive impact on fauna." *Ann N Y Acad Sci.* 2009;1181:255–80.

Yan C, Boyd DD. "Histone H3 acetylation and H3 K4 methylation define distinct chromatin regions permissive for transgene expression." *Mol Cell Biol.* 2006;26(17):6357–71.

Yu CC, et al. "Genome-wide DNA methylation and gene expression analyses of monozygotic twins discordant for intelligence levels." *PLoS One.* 2012;7(10).

Zhang X, et al. "Genome-wide study of DNA methylation alterations in response to diazinon exposure in vitro." *Environ Toxicol Pharmacol.* 2012;34(3):959–68.

Zöchbauer-Müller S, Minna JD, Gazdar AF. "Aberrant DNA methylation in lung cancer: biological and clinical implications." *Oncologist.* 2002;7(5): 451–7.

Index

Numbers in **bold italics** indicate pages with photographs.

Index

Baccarelli, A. 201*n*20
bacterial species 148
Bakulski, K.M. 192*n*15, 192*n*16
Barile, F.A. 192*n*18
bases 11
Baskin-Robbins 33
Batelle 185*n*5, 203*n*3
Baylin, Dr. Stephen 71
BDNF 127
Beatles 191*n*20
Beijing 116
Bell labs 173
bell shaped curve *158*, 202*n*10
benzene 73, 178
Berlin 88
Bernal, A.L. 200*n*6
Berns, G. 188*ch*4*n*4
beta amyloid 98
beta cells 82
BioIT World 185*n*10
biomonitoring 92
Biopharm International 202*n*13
biopharma company 67
biosphere 149
bipolar disorder 1, 108–110, 127, 168–169
Bird, S.C. 185*n*2
birds 147–148
Birnbaum, L.S. 196*n*18
birth control pills 201*n*17
birth defect 54, 125, 187*n*2
bisphenol A 91, 163, 190*n*21, 191*n*16,
    191*n*17, 191*n*18, 191*n*19, 191*n*20, 200*n*7,
    200*n*13
Blackett, Piers R. 81, 190*n*1
blastema 198*n*8
blastocyst *16*, 19
blastula 13
blindness 81
blood pressure 126
blood sugar 86
Blue Brain Project 117, 195*n*7
The Blue Danube Waltz 117
Blumenthal, T. 185*n*13
Boehner, John 153, 201*n*6, 202*n*6
Bohacek, J. 194*n*6
Bollati, V. 201*n*20
Bortone, S.A. 200*n*15
Bota, S. 189*n*8
Bouchard, T.J., Jr. 196*n*13
boxing 100, 192*n*9; ban on 100, 192*n*11
Boyd, D.D. 185*n*9
The Boys from Brazil 15
BPA 76, 79, 90, 92–94, 145, 147–151,
    199*n*2, 199*n*6

BPS 151
brain 100–101, 118, 131; atrophy 87; cells
    109, 116; disorders 203*n*1; function 122;
    trauma 100
"The Brains of the Animal Kingdom"
    188*ch*4*n*4
BRCA1 70
BRCA2 70
breast epithelial cells 76
Brenner, D.J. 186*n*7
Brewer, G.L. 104, 193*n*23
Bridges, Calvin 186*n*5
Briggs, R. 14, 184*n*9
Brno in Moravia 10
Brody, Adrian 26
bronchial 189*n*8
bronchoscopy 64
Brown, A. 203*n*20
Bulgaria 73, 189*n*18
Buxhoeveden, D.P. 195*n*6
bytes 95

cadmium 76, 102
caffeine 143–144, 199*n*3
California 123, 131
Calment, Jeanne 132, 197*n*3
caloric restriction 164
The Caloric Restriction Society 190*n*9,
    191*n*9
Cameron, J.A. 198*n*8
Canada 93, 154
cancer 1, 3, 23, 39, 41, 44–46, 48, 57,
    60–61, 63–65, 68–70, 75, 87, 106, 131–
    132, 144, 160, 162, 167–168, 171, 188*n*2,
    204*n*3; bladder 74, 77; breast 70, 162;
    cells 42, 64; cervical 62, 71; colon 72;
    environmentally-based 80; epigenetic
    78; kidney 70, 72; lung 63, 74, 77, 162,
    203*n*18; management 189*n*9; ovarian
    70; prostate 62–63; rates of 77; stom-
    ach 68, 189*n*12; surgery 59; treatment
    42; vaccine 63; War on 61
"Cancer Research UK" 188*n*6
Carboniferous period 39
carcinogen 45, 60, 75, 167, 199*n*5
carcinoma 188*n*1
Cardiff 59
cardiology 196*n*5
cardiovascular disease 30, 82, 87, 91, 101,
    132, 134, 168
Carlson, E.A. 186*n*3
Carlsson, H.E. 187*n*3
Carnes, B.A. 198*n*17, 199*n*20
Carson, Rachel 200*n*16

212